Moon Time

Cover design by Lucy Pearce

Layout by Treacy-Pearce Solutions

Cover image: © Leziles | Dreamstime.com

All images are author's own work, except those detailed below:

Moon dial mandala created by Zoe Shekinah (p.49)

NIGHT YOGA (p.82)
© Ivan Hafizov | Dreamstime.com

ROSE IN HAIR (p.102)
© Agnieszka Pastuszak - Maksim | Dreamstime.com

PEACEFUL DRINK (p.116)
© Nitipong Ballapavanich | Dreamstime.com

Extended quotations used with the express permission of their authors.

The herbal and nutritional advice contained in this book is provided as information, not formal medical advice. It is recommended that you seek further professional advice before following it.

ISBN: 1468056719
ISBN-13: 978-1468056716

"This book is a wonderful journey of discovery. Lucy not only guides us through the wisdom inherent in our wombs, our cycles and our hearts, but also encourages us to share, express, celebrate and enjoy what it means to be female!

A beautiful and inspiring book full of practical information and ideas."

Miranda Gray, author *Red Moon* and *The Optimized Woman*

OOO

"Lucy, your book, Moon Time, is monumental. I cannot tell you how long I have thought of the very things you are putting forward, and to see this in print is thrilling.

Moon Time is a well needed resource book covering a wide range of important ways to respect our blood cycles wisely. Holding our cycles, bodies, and stages in life with the highest regard breaks the spell of centuries of oppression where our blood has been considered a dirty curse. The wisdom in Moon Time sets a new course where we glimpse a future culture reshaped by honoring our womanhood journeys one woman at a time.

Cozy up, get yourself a cup of tea and come home as a daughter of the Red River flowing."

ALisa Starkweather, founder of Red Tent Temple Movement. Contributing author to *Women, Spirituality and Transformative Leadership: Where Grace Meets Power.*

"Lucy Pearce weaves a moon-web that draws in the many other women who have written on the subject of menstrual cycles and places herself as one, amongst others. Her open and accessible book offers practical, often humorous ideas and encouragement about how we can tune into our own cycles and 'dance' with them in the most creative and healthy way.

She is one of the special whisperers, who helps us to remember our own power and sacredness as played out in our cycles. Through her writing she initiates a dialogue with her readers. Her writing empowers her readers to have a voice to respond. This is a remarkable gift to us."

Tracy Evans, MA researcher, women's rites of passage, University of Aberystwyth

OOO

"Moon Time is a beautifully written resource for deepening your connection with your cycle. Full of personal heartfelt suggestions, simple rituals and practical ways to support women in understanding the influence their hormones have on them each month.

This book could change your life!"

Rachael Hertogs, compiling editor of *Thirteen Moons* and author *Menarche: A Journey to Womanhood*

Moon Time

ooo

A guide to celebrating
your menstrual cycle

Lucy H. Pearce

OOO

For my mother:

I am me,

Because you were you.

OOO

CONTENTS

ACKNOWLEDGEMENTS

I wish to thank all those who have supported my writing and my life as they have unfolded:

My mother, Francesca, for giving me life, and making me who I am.

My father, Stephen, for providing the template for making a living from honouring your creativity. And for creating and sharing the tea house where this book was written.

My grandmothers, Lucy and Suzanne, who shaped me more than they could possibly know, and whose physical presence I miss deeply, but whose spirits are always by my side.

My step-mother, Lauren: part mother, part sister, part friend, but as far from wicked as it's possible to get!

My sister Mirin, for blossoming into the young woman I always wished I had been, right in front of my eyes.

My best school friend, Emma, with whom I shared the news of my first bleeding and the joy of my first birth, as well as many other secrets along the way.

My women's group: Amy, Meadhbh, Delphine, Louise, Mary, Leigh and Loo for holding the container of our collective womb within which we have all grown.

My soul sisters: Tracy, Mary, Leigh, Laura and Paula. For seeing me as I am – and celebrating that with me.

My moon dancing sister in America, Becky Jaine – shine on!

My treasured readers at Dreaming Aloud and Juno for their unfailing enthusiasm and positive feedback over the years. A writer is nothing without her readers.

ALisa, Miranda, Rachael, Nicholas, Isadora, Shawn, Zoe and Dawn for their beautiful work which inspired me, and their generous, open-hearted permission to reproduce it in this book. Your blessings for my work have touched my soul.

My husband, Patrick, for his technical prowess – everything I don't know how to do, he does – we make a good team! For supporting my women's work and creativity, for being open to sharing working and childcare, for keeping me sane and helping me to laugh over the years, I am incredibly grateful. You truly are my soft place to fall.

And finally to our three children: Timmy, Merrily and Aisling, for their patience with me when the Crazy Woman roams, my distractedness when a creative project is gestating, as well as for their love and the fun that we share. I am so glad to be your mother.

INTRODUCTION

At her first bleeding a woman meets her power.

During her bleeding years she practices it.

At menopause she becomes it.

Traditional Native American saying

Welcome dearest woman.

I am so glad you could join me. It is my deepest wish to help you to celebrate your female rhythms so that you can find balance in your life.

It is my guess that no one ever initiated you into the path of womanhood. Instead, just like me, you were left to find out by yourself. Little by little you pieced a working understanding of your body and soul together.

But still you yearn for a greater knowledge, an understanding of who you are, why you are that way, and how you can learn to ride your female cycles with grace and ease.

Perhaps you have searched long and hard, seeking advice from your mother, sister, aunts and friends. Perhaps they were not to be spoken of at home. You may have visited doctors, healers or therapists, but still you feel at sea in the mystery of your woman's body.

Or maybe you have never given your cycles a second thought…until now.

So here we are, sat together, over a steaming cup of herbal tea. Allow the questions that you have to bubble up. What is your experience of being a woman like right now? How would you like it to be? What do you need?

Perhaps you are seeking…

o   deeper harmony with yourself and your cycle

o   greater self-knowledge and self-acceptance

o   an understanding of your fertility

o   rituals to express your feminine creativity

o   an enhanced relationship with your family at "that time of the month"

o   a way to balance your hectic life and your body's needs

o   healing for past hurts to do with starting your period

o   positive language to describe your body and its functions

o   a guide to creating a red tent or moon lodge

o   natural ways of dealing with PMT

o   support in celebrating your daughter's impending womanhood

o   a greater connection to nature's cycles, seasons and the moon

o   a deeper connection with other women

o   healthy, happy menstruation

Introduction

In this guide I will share with you:

o   creative tools to help you celebrate your cycle

o   rituals for self-care

o   nutritional and herbal suggestions for supporting you through your cycle

o   spiritual/ wise woman insight into your cycle.

Learning to celebrate your cyclical nature will naturally lead to a greater sense of ease, well-being, physical and emotional comfort.

Through knowledge we gain power over our lives.

With options we have possibility.

With acceptance we find a new freedom.

Not everything here might be for you now at this point in your journey. Perhaps you are just beginning the journey of self-acceptance, just starting to learn about your body's cycles. Or perhaps you have been studying them for years and are wanting resources to help you dig deeper into yourself, to empower you to share your journey and wisdom with other women in your community.

Whatever your starting point, whatever your background I want this to be deeply accessible and acceptable to you, so that you can move deeper into your own wisdom and begin to:

o   learn to trust that your body and its functions hold immense power and wisdom

o   own what you know

o   understand that knowing goes beyond thoughts and the brain

o   be true to yourself

o   commit to self-care.

So if I suggest something which doesn't sit well with you, I invite you to examine it:

o   is it uncomfortable to you simply because it is a new idea?

o   is it something you have been taught to reject or disapprove of?

o   is it something which you feel others might judge you on or ridicule?

o   is it something you have tried and know you don't like?

o   or are we coming from different assumptions or understandings?

To thine own self be true

As you work through this book, be true to yourself, follow your own inner compass, whilst gently opening your heart and mind. So if I suggest dancing, and you hate to dance, then think – what is the alternative? What feels right to me? Or if I suggest incense or herbs and that's not your thing, that is completely fine. These are things that have worked for me and other women. But maybe they're just not for you. What is **your** thing?

I do not want you to change one iota of yourself, unless of course you want to.

You are perfect, exactly as you are, right now!

Lighting all the incense in the world isn't going to put you in touch with your female cycles. Pretending to be someone you're not leads you away from self-knowledge. And so, whilst this book contains Native American wisdom, I am not expecting you to become a Red Indian. Nor an ancient Canaanite or a raving hippy for that matter! You are you. And that is as it should be.

Consider this a bag of seeds. You choose which to plant, and when and where. You are the gardener of your own life. Follow your own path to self-knowledge by focusing on what is in your heart, and listening to what your body is telling you. That is the key. This book offers you hundreds of different ways in. All it takes is one to start you on your own path, or unblock the way.

Introduction

With much of this women's work, because it goes against the grain of what we have been taught in our culture, many of us find that it is easier to start small and private, whilst we are still learning and growing. Just as we would protect a small precious seedling from being eaten or trampled by wild animals.

Each step, each learning, is a step closer to blossoming into your full knowledge and woman's wisdom.

It is a long path, a spiral path, around to the dark side of the moon and back into the light, cycle after cycle, for our whole reproductive lives and beyond.

Take your time.

Be gentle with yourself.

Remember that you are not alone. All around the world, over two billion women are travelling this path: silent sisters of the moon. Through this book you will learn how to kindle your own wisdom flame, and share it together with your daughters and sisters. You will find ways to celebrate and support each other, and begin to break our silence – if you feel called to.

So here we are, at the beginning of our journey together, to explore the mystery of being a woman.

Enter with me, in the spirit of self-love. Let us transform and celebrate our moon time together.

OOO

My own journey

I always find it helps on a journey, to know a little about my companion and where she has come from, so that we can travel in trust and ease together.

I am a home-birth mama to three children (now aged 6,3 and 1). I have been working in sacred women's work for the past five years, running women's circles, mother blessing ceremonies and holistic birth preparation classes. I am working to set up my own red tent here in East Cork. I write on women's issues (natural pregnancy, birth, motherhood, moon time and health) in my career as a free-spirited, freelance writer, blogger and contributing editor at JUNO magazine.

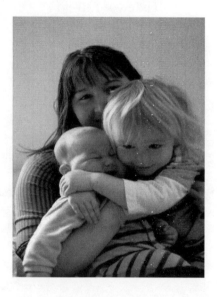

Whilst many of my credentials are quite alternative, I am not, if truth be told, that comfortable with anything too "out there". And so, the thrust of my work is, and always has been, to bring the wisdom of the alternative movement back into the mainstream, to make it accessible to all.

For me the transition to awareness about myself as a woman happened as a result of gestating, birthing and breastfeeding three children. There is nothing like being caught in this cycle of procreation for seven years to put one in touch with one's body and how it works!

Coming back to my periods after prolonged breaks each time gave me a chance to be more reflective and aware of them rather than simply reacting to them. I was aware from first-hand experience of the power of my womb to create, hold and give birth to life. I understood its function. The point of periods was no longer abstract, and my sexuality was not just fun, or limited by fear of pregnancy. A greater sense of gratitude and compassion for myself and all women came with this embodied knowing of the function and wisdom of my womb and ovaries and the intricate chemical dance of my hormones, which goes on unseen by me.

Rather than force myself to be like a man, I understood that I really am a woman. I really do have many different moods to my physical and emotional life, and so I have learnt to celebrate them rather than ignore them. To co-create with them rather than resist them. And this truly has been a wonderful journey, which I want to share with you.

It was when I was twenty, struggling with being on the Pill and hating it, that I came across the book *Women's Bodies, Women's Wisdom* which set me on a path of curiosity and discovery about my own female body.

Fast forward more than a decade, and I realised that at 31 years old, I am already more than halfway through my moon journey. And though I have read and researched women's wisdom, and bled for twenty years, I am only just starting to fully embrace my own embodied female wisdom and apply it.

I feel like a slow learner! But then I look around me and almost all the women I know of my age, and older, are in this place of only beginning their learning.

We are not initiated into what it means to become a woman.

We were not taught this... so why should we know?

OOO

The lessons of the Western world

(Why not tick off those which you have been taught!)

o   Our cycles are not of any relevance or importance to us or our world.

o   Women are unreliable and too emotional because of their periods.

o   It is preferable to avoid menstruation. It is a problem which most women would like to be rid of.

o   It is a topic for smutty jokes and mockery about 'being on the rag'.

o   Periods prevent us from being fully functional or rational, and so unable to play roles of importance in a man's world.

o   Menstruation is embarrassing and dirty.

o   Hide it away, don't talk about it; be silent and discrete.

o   If you experience discomfort seek out a doctor to help you silence your symptoms.

o   Don't get pregnant! (Until you're 30).

o   Or why can't you get pregnant? (If you're over 30).

o   Mothering is not an important or valued role.

OOO

Throughout the book you will find "And you…" sections which invite you to reflect and respond, to apply what you have read to yourself. Perhaps you would like to note answers to the questions briefly in your journal. Perhaps some call you to a longer, more detailed response. Or maybe you just want to answer them in your head as you read. As with the rest of this book, do what works for you!

And you...

Which of these lessons are true for you?

Are there any more lessons that you would add?

Which of these do you still believe or live by

Which have you rejected?

What were you taught about being a cycling woman – by whom?

Was it explicitly taught or merely implied?

How do you feel about your cycles at the moment?

How has this evolved over the years?

There is little understanding and allowance for the realities of being a cycling woman, let alone celebration.

But that changes here!

Take my hand...

Let us begin!

1

OUR CYCLES
A BIOLOGICAL UNDERSTANDING

A woman re-dreams the world when she bleeds.

Native American wisdom

Whilst most of us learned about our female biology in school science classes, this was usually from a detached perspective – full of big scientific words and abstract diagrams – which often felt like it had little to do with us.

We are not taught in school about the experiential aspects of our cycles, or the spiritual and intuitive gifts of menstruation. When we understand what is happening inside we can learn how to live our lives in harmony with this, rather than fighting or ignoring our biology.

Menstruation

We start bleeding earlier than at the beginning of the twentieth century, with girls' first periods occurring at 12.8 years, compared with14.5 years. Coupled with lower breastfeeding rates, better nutrition, and fewer pregnancies, women now menstruate more in their adult lives than ever before.

"Each month a woman's body undergoes a series of changes, many of which occur without her being consciously aware of them. These include variations in hormone balances, vaginal temperature, uterine composition and quantity, body weight, vitamin concentrations, water retention, heart rate, breast size and consistency, concentration levels, vision and hearing, psychic ability, pain threshold and many others."
Miranda Gray, *Red Moon*

The changes are most definitely not "all in your head" as many would have us believe. This is why it is so crucial to honour these changes by adapting our lives to them as much as possible.

We cannot just will these changes not to happen as they are an integral part of our fertility.

To ensure that we all share the same basic understanding of what is actually happening inside our bodies, this chapter provides a quick overview of the biology of our cycles. For a more in depth understanding I recommend Toni Weschler's *Taking Charge of Your Fertility* or Dr Christiane Northrup's *Women's Bodies, Women's Wisdom.*

Menstruation

o   **Day 1** is the first day of bleeding. The bleeding occurs when the nutrient rich womb lining disintegrates and is shed because no egg has been implanted.

o   This usually lasts 4-6 days getting lighter in the final couple of days.

o   Only an egg-cup full of blood is lost, but it looks like a lot more!

o   If you are taking the Pill, the bleeding that you experience is not a menstrual period but simply a withdrawal bleed from the artificially induced state of quasi-pregnancy that the hormones create.

Pre-ovulation

o   Oestrogen increases leading to the development of the egg follicles and stimulation of the breast and uterine wall.

Ovulation

o   At ovulation time (around day 12-16) usually just one egg is released from one of your fallopian tubes (they alternate each month).

o   You will notice a change in your discharge around this time. You will most likely feel very wet, and your underwear will be damp from the discharge which is clear and stretchy like egg white. It can often feel like you have just got your period. You will most likely feel sexier. If you are wanting to get pregnant, now's the time!

o   The egg becomes a corpus luteum producing both oestrogen and progesterone in preparation for fertilisation.

Pre-menstrual phase

o   The pre-menstrual stage can last for up to a week before bleeding starts.

o   If fertilisation does not occur the corpus luteum degenerates and the levels of progesterone and oestrogen both fall.

o   This change in hormones can lead to PMS symptoms.

o   Most women have a second window of sexual excitement either just before or towards the end of menstruation.

o   There is a biological need for increased REM (dreaming) sleep from day 25 onwards.

Many women have regular cycles of around 28 days, though others might have cycles of varying lengths (14-40 days), and periods of varying lengths (3-7 days). What is most important is that you know what "normal" is for you.

Some women naturally have shorter or longer cycles their whole lives, however if:

o   your periods are very irregular,

o   you have a lot of mid-cycle spotting,

o   your period is very light (pale pink and watery),

o   it is extremely heavy,

o   it contains lots of clots,

o   PMT symptoms are incapacitating,

o   you are struggling to conceive,

I do recommend that you visit a practitioner – perhaps an acupuncturist or herbalist – to help you to establish a rhythm. This is especially important if you are wanting to chart your cycles either to avoid pregnancy or to find out your peak fertile time.

Irregular cycles and the other issues mentioned are often symptomatic of an underlying health issue which needs to be addressed such as a hormonal imbalance, nutritional deficiency, weight issues, emotional stress or being generally run-down.

Menstruation and breastfeeding

There is little common knowledge about the interaction between menstruation and lactation, perhaps because at the time when much of the scientific research on menstruation was happening in the West, breastfeeding levels were at their lowest since humans' emergence on this planet.

o   Prolactin, the major hormone which enables breastfeeding, supresses fertility. However, only whilst the baby is being fed every two hours during the day and at least twice a night, and is exclusively breastfed. This natural pause to the cycles is called lactational amenorrhea.
o   Extended periods of lactational amenorrhea result in lower rates of breast, ovarian and endometrial cancers.
o   Fertility may re-appear anything from four weeks after birth to over three years. With mothers who breastfeed exclusively, it is usually over six months, and often over a year.
o   The first periods may occur without ovulation, but equally fertility might reappear without menstruation, and with no obvious signs to alert you.
o   It is completely possible to conceive whilst breastfeeding. However, some women might need to cut down feeds or stop feeding all together to ensure a return to full fertility.
o   Chinese medicine states that bleeding and lactating both deplete the body, and do not recommend doing both. If you are, then it is vital that you support your system with optimum nutrition, extra rest and perhaps herbs.

o   Readjusting to your menstrual cycles after pregnancy and feeding can be a gradual process, with periods taking a while to establish their regular rhythm.

o   Return to menstruation can be accompanied by emotional upheaval including: grief, depression, exhaustion, it may also bring renewed energy and a feeling of "being back to yourself".

Menopause

Menopause refers to the last menstrual period. It occurs at some point between 40 and 55 years, with the average being 51 years. It is considered conclusive when you have 12 months without a period.

o   Pre-menopause can last 10 years. During this time the ovaries gradually stop maturing eggs and releasing large amounts of hormones.

o   Peri-menopause refers to the few years before and one year after the final period where symptoms are usually apparent.

o   Menopausal symptoms include: hot flushes, night sweats, mood swings, vaginal dryness and irregular periods.

o   Bleeding becomes lighter, or sometimes much heavier, and changes in frequency as ovulation becomes more sporadic.

OOO

For many of us this basic biological understanding is where our education about our female bodies stopped. But there is so much more to learn! So let us delve deeper into what it means to be a cycling woman. Let us examine the intricate interweaving of our bodies, hormones and psyches which make us the women we are. Let us come home to ourselves in all our complexity and embrace our ever-changing selves, the light and darkness both. Let us meet ourselves with open arms and understanding, with creativity and curiosity

.

2

OUR CYCLES
ARCHETYPAL INSIGHT

*By being true to all sides of your nature, you acknowledge that
you can be self-confident, active and strong, that you can nurture
without being weak, that you can be wild and instinctual as well
as calm and reasoning, and that you have a beautiful darkness
within, a depth beyond the mundane world.*

Miranda Gray, *Red Moon*

The wisdom of our cycles works on every level. Through our cycles our
bodies regenerate their life-giving ability. During our moon time we dive into
our depths, mining gems of intuitive wisdom. And in the mid- part of our
cycles we are gifted with the energy to bring these forth – to birth our gifts,
our children and our creations into the world.

Our cycles ensure that we do not live static lives. Instead they demand that we
live dynamically, constantly exploring the different gifts of feminine power

which each portion of our cycle holds. Part of learning the art of being a woman is learning to honour each element of our cycles and ourselves.

A woman's cycle takes her each month on a journey between the light and dark parts of her soul. When she is unskilled or unprepared, she may stumble, falling over her own feet and everything that lies in her path.

As she gains confidence in herself and senses her own rhythms she begins to dance to her own tune. She gains mastery over her own body: she is coordinated and graceful. She can sense when too increase her energetic output. As her internal rhythm becomes juicy, vibrant and abundant and sexually alluring she swirls and leaps in pure joy and abundance.

Then the stormy part of the symphony emerges – she swoops and stamps, tears and grasps. The cymbals crash, the drums crescendo.

And then the music begins to quieten, she strains to hear, she slows her movements, she is elegant and restrained. Her gestures are more subtle, stilled almost to silence, her dance has moved inside. From the twitch of her hand, the glow in her eye you can see the inner dance progress.

The music begins to rise and so does she – up from the ground where she has lain, new-born, her movements are light and fresh, dainty, gaining confidence and momentum as her sap rises, the moon rises and she leaps to hold it in her arms once more.

Our cycles have four major phases, which can be interpreted as corresponding to the four main female archetypes (or energy patterns) and stages of life.

The Virgin/Maiden

The virgin self emerges after the menstrual bleeding has stopped, and the fresh new womb lining grows. This phase is seen as the phase of the virgin.

She is full of innocence, energy and potential. She feels good in her body – flirtatious, sexy and lighter after the dark days of her blood time. Her ability to conceive and gestate are just emerging, and are still unproven. At his point in her cycle, she feels freest from her menstrual pull – she is a virgin in the traditional sense of the word – a woman unto herself.

The Mother

The time of ovulation and possible conception is represented by the mother who has the ability to nurture new life. Her fertile womb space is warm and soft. At this time a woman tends to feel loving and enjoys giving of herself fully, either by becoming a mother to a child, or in her career, creativity or home making. Ovulation symbolises the ability to give and sustain life and the full flourishing of a woman's life.

The Enchantress/ Wild Woman

The pre-menstrual stage is a descent from the light, outward stage of our cycle and into the dark, inner stage. Progesterone and oestrogen dance together to create dynamic swings. The wild woman dances a magical path between huge bouts of creativity and emotional storms. In becoming a wise woman you learn how to harness this powerful energy, knowing when to destroy, how to express your righteous anger, and when to go within and reflect.

The Crone/ Wise Woman

The crone emerges during the late pre-menstrual and bleeding time. She can be a wise woman or a destructive witch depending on how she handles this time. Her mood darkens and she becomes pulled inward, becoming quieter, more reflective and more in touch with the dream time. She is less "in the world" and like an older person is in need of more rest. This time has many gifts for the woman and her community, if she can learn to retreat and allow her visions to emerge from her darkest depths.

OOO

We live in a culture which worships the virgin, her nubile body and budding sexuality. One which side-lines the mother, not celebrating or honouring the acts of gestation, birth and childrearing. A culture which fears the power of the enchantress, which turns away from the wisdom of the elders and does not know the value of reflection and dreams.

In order to reclaim our full selves, to integrate each of these aspects through which we will pass into our lives, we must first learn to embrace them though our cycles.

We need to take time to honour the part of ourselves which mothers and nurtures; the part of us which yearns to be girlish and free; the wise woman who watches in the wings full of wisdom and the erotic enchantress who can bewitch and create magic. Our cycles allow us to take on these roles, to live these hidden parts of our psyches – perhaps they are stages we have already passed through in our lives, glad that they are behind us, or sad for their loss, or stages we feel uncomfortable with becoming.

Our cycling nature gives us constant teasing tastes of the whole gamut of womanhood, and our life cycle, month after month. It also ensures that we deal with emotions which we might otherwise avoid: anger, sadness, conflict, grief and eroticism.

We are always much more complex, much wiser than we give ourselves credit for, our potential much greater than we dare to hope or dream.

OOO

Living and working by our cycles

"With the encroachment of the female into the "male world", the advancement of women has been mostly intellectual, empty of the intuitive understanding and creative which is the basis of their nature. There are no archetypes or traditions to guide women on their needs and abilities in these new modern areas of work and experience. It is therefore vitally important that women redress this lack, that they take their awareness of their cyclic nature into the workplace and general

community, help society to see it as a positive and empowering force on all levels – at work, in business, in the family, in relationships, in education, in medicine, and in creating personal growth and goals – and that they help to build guidelines, approaches and new traditions for women to follow."

Miranda Gray, *Red Moon*

Depending your work and living situation, you will have greater or lesser flexibility to link your work and daily rhythm to your cycle.

But we all have some power over our days, although learning to exercise this, and voice our needs, or to actively set the rhythm we need, can be hugely challenging to many women. But know that you, and all around you, will reap the rewards, as you become more productive, creative and healthy. Please be aware that the suggestions below are general guidelines. Through growing awareness of your own physical and emotional cues, which you will gain by charting, you will recognise and learn to live by your own unique rhythms.

"The traditional, linear view of a period of time – say a year – could be described as a series of jobs or projects, each of which will be carried through with times of high input and low input until they are completed. If you view the year as a series of repeating cycles, it should be possible to arrange the tasks so that each receives the most appropriate attention and energy at each phase in your cycle."

Miranda Gray, *Red Moon*

Pre-ovulation

You will most probably be feeling calm, open, dynamic, clear, energetic and enthusiastic. You will have the capacity for high levels of mental and physical activity. Start by catching up with things that may have slipped during menstruation. This is the time to start projects: organise and prioritise your time and energy to get the best results. Make to-do lists and tick off all that you achieve.

This is a great time for a clear out as you have lots of energy and little emotional attachment to things – now is the time for spring cleaning. Any fresh starts you need to make in your life: instigating healthy eating or exercise regimes, or searching for a partner. Do it now!

Ovulation

The motto for this time of your cycle is "work hard, love well." Give birth to creative projects that you have been gestating. This is the time to stay up late – but be careful not to burn out by trying to be superwoman – you will pay for it later in the cycle!

You may feel attuned to other women, especially mothers, and generally receptive to others' input. Now is a great time for team work and collaboration. Now is also the time when you can get pregnant – so be careful, or go for it, depending on your intentions!

Take advantage of your nurturing energy to visit family and friends who you find demanding. Indulge your mothering side with your own children if you have them.

Turn your attention to making your home feel welcoming and full of love. Have friends over or entertain work colleagues. If you can, fill your freezer and larder with food that you have made to see you through the hungry gap of your late cycle when you will probably not feel like cooking. This nourishing food will make all the difference and will stop you snacking on junk which makes PMT symptoms worse.

Pre-menstrual

Start to cut back on work which requires collaboration or high levels of energy. Do not plan athletic or endurance events for this time. Try to avoid long, tiring journeys, especially across time zones.

This is the time for dealing with frustrations and irritations – but only if you can allow yourself to interact with a modicum of reason as well as powerful emotion! Do not be too hasty, pick fights or burn your bridges at a whim at this time – it is easily done! Instead take notes on your feelings, tell a friend or partner, allow them to be a sounding board before you take decisive action.

Now is the time to go into planning and evaluation mode. Focus on administration, sedentary activities, project work which does not require too much concentration or fine motor skills. Allow yourself more sleep and early nights. Avoid evening meetings or late night parties as your moon time approaches and avoid encounters which are liable to make you overly emotional. Now is the time to try more personal creative projects which require intuitive guidance and reflection.

Menstruation

If you can take a day or two at the start of your menstruation to retreat then do. Later in this book I will share tools for creating your own retreat space. Perhaps you can only manage a couple of hours in the evening to yourself – then make that a priority – put it in your diary just as you would with any other important appointment.

If you can cut back your hours and make them up later in the month, then do. Perhaps you can work from home or hire someone to help. Cut back to absolute minimum for 3-5 days (ideally two days pre-menstrually and for the first three days of your period). Use this time to dream, rest, reflect, evaluate. Work by yourself as much as possible. If you have simple repetitive tasks which need doing, now is the time for sedentary activities, ones which do not require too much of your concentration. Do not take any big decisions. Let me repeat, do not put yourself under pressure to make decisions! Take a long lunch. Eat nourishing food. Stay warm.

Cycles within cycles

It is important to note that within our monthly (moon influenced) and daily (sun influenced) cycles we also have "ultradians", meaning cycles which recur regularly many times throughout the day. Dr Ernest Rossi discovered that we have periods of 1½ hours of alertness and focus followed by 20 minutes of required rest or downtime, to ensure optimum functioning. It is vitally important to honour this rhythm throughout your menstrual cycle – on days of high energy and low. And whilst you may not be able to have a complete break, ensure that you take a couple of minutes to stretch, walk, yawn, go outside, close your eyes, have a drink or snack at these regular intervals throughout the day – just listen to your body's signals, it will tell you what you need.

OOO

Menstruation and fertility

Our periods are often looked at in isolation from our fertility and feelings about fertility. In my own personal experience, and that of women that I know, how we feel about getting pregnant majorly impacts our attitudes towards our moon time and our bodies.

Virgin

For younger women who dread the inconvenience of pregnancy, and just desire to be free and easy in their bodies, like they were as a pre-teen and as boys their age are, a period is a major inconvenience to be ignored. This is the time when we often go on the Pill, use tampons and struggle with the worst elements of PMT – the monthly hormones exacerbating teenage issues like acne, body issues, greasy hair and mood swings. This is a time when we neither value nor desire our fertility, and therefore often reject our periods.

Mother

For women wanting to get pregnant but who are struggling, a period often means a failure, the lack of fertility, and with it brings grief, anger and despair, thus exacerbating PMT.

For a woman who is breastfeeding, the return of her cycles means extra tiredness to her already overused body, a sense of being swamped by a baby when she needs space to bleed. It also means the return of the anxiety about fertility, and if and when another baby is desired.

Enchantress

For women who have given birth and are reasonably at peace with their family size, many of these issues are gone and the monthly period gives a reminder of the miracle of the bodily cycles which helped to create her children. But it also creates a time of disharmony when she is required to care for children and needs to retreat.

Crone

For an older woman, each missed period gives a reminder that her years of fertility are behind her and that a new stage of life awaits. It may be the first time that her sexuality is totally unfettered by her fertility. But it can also be an unwelcome reminder that she is ageing. The way that she perceives older women and death can impact her experiences profoundly.

OOO

Integrated menstrual chart

I have compiled the information from the past two chapters: biological, archetypal, spiritual and emotional, into a simple chart format, condensing the ideas into a clear reference tool.

You could photocopy it and keep in your journal or pin on the wall by your desk as a reminder of your ever-changing self. You could illustrate it, colour it or laminate it…

It is yours to use in the way that supports you best. My deepest wish is that it will guide you in your journey of self-discovery.

You will find a full-colour version to download for yourself or share with your friends on my website www.thehappywomb.com

Phase	Pre ovulatory	Ovulatory
Moon phase	Waxing	Full
Archetype	Virgin/ Maiden	Mother
Season	Spring	Summer
Element	Air	Earth
Light	Lightening	Full bright light
Length	9 days	5 days
Hormone	Oestrogen	Rising oestrogen and progesterone
Physical	Egg follicle ripening – stimulating breast and womb	Egg released from ovary into fallopian tube, becomes 'corpus luteum'. Uterine wall built up in preparation for fertilisation
Vaginal Discharge	Sticky/ none	Clear and stretchy, like egg white. Very wet feeling
Emotion	Calm, open, dynamic, clear, energetic, enthusiastic, able to cope with irritations	Loving, nurturing, nourishing, sustaining, energised, connected
Energy	Rising dynamic – growing outward	Full, sustaining – losing sense of self in work or mothering

Pre-menstrual	Menstrual
Waning	Dark
Enchantress/ Wild Woman	Crone/ Wise Woman
Autumn	Winter
Fire	Water
Darkening	Dark
9 days	5 days
Falling oestrogen and progesterone	Progesterone
Transition time	Womb lining breaks down and released from uterus
None/ blobby thick and yellow	Bleeding – starting out bright red, becoming browner towards the end
Creative, emotional, sensitive	Introspective, dreamy, sensitive, intuitive, spiritually connected
Waning dynamic – destructive, descending inward	Reflective, slow, containing, internalised, spiritual

Libido	Rising – carefree	Full, horny, height of libidinous desire around full moon/ ovulation
Physical feeling	Energetic	Perhaps ovulatory pain/ cramping, sometimes mid cycle spotting, food cravings, horny, sensitive breasts
Outward action	Start projects – clear visioning and energy raising. Fresh start. Organise and prioritise. Clear out – spring cleaning. Catch up with things that have slipped during menstruation	Work hard, love well – birth creative projects, stay up late! Harmony with nature and other mothers. Receptive to other's input
Relationships	Easy-going, trusting, out going	Loving, giving, nurturing. Reach out to friends, children, family and partner
Key words	New beginnings, dynamic, exuberance, self-confident	Fertility, radiating, caring, nurturing, committed
Affirmation	I step forward in action with a lightness of heart	I embrace my life with love and generate beauty around me

Peaks and troughs – can be very intense	Often a sexual peak just before bleeding occurs, or just after. Little desire during menstruation
Lowered immune system. Towards the end cramping, back ache, bloating, tiredness, tender breasts, sugar and carbohydrate cravings, hostility, mood swings	Greater need for rest and dreaming sleep. Cramping, back ache, migraine, faintness, exhaustion, tearfulness
Finish up projects. Begin to reflect and assess. Take action dealing with issues and problems	Retreat, dream time. Only do what is essential. Do not take on any new projects. Delay important decisions or stressful appointments
Turn your focus to inner-directed creative projects and listen deeply to your intuition	Slow down, tune in deeply to your intuition and rest well
Needs to balance dynamic interactions with others, with focused, energised creative time alone	Desires to be alone or in quiet communion with other women – does not want to be around men and children!
Magical, witchy, destructive, intuitive	Darkness, wisdom, gestation, stillness, vision
I use the sword of my intolerance to cut deep and true. I keep hold of my vision and manifest it	I sink into my depths and listen to my dreams

Visualising your archetypes

If the idea of archetypes (Maiden, Mother, Enchantress and Wise Woman) speaks to you, then why not bring them to life for yourself? The following exercise will help you to integrate their different energies further into your life. The exercise is divided into a couple of stages – the first step is visualising the associations you have with each of the archetypes, the second is representing them creatively.

You do not need to be a professional artist to have a go! It is about building your understanding of the different energies as represented by the archetypal characters. Your intention needs to be expressing the basic energy of each phase of the cycle – your representations do not need to be "perfect", they are your personal expressions of your personal understanding. If you really, really freak out at the idea of putting brush to paper, then just do this as an active visualisation, taking yourself through the steps in your mind's eye.

This project can take place over the course of a month. Or it could be a moon time project. I recommend that you choose one medium (i.e. paint, pastel, clay) to create the whole series, so that you have a complete cycle and you can see how the energy alters the identical materials.

Take what you learn from it and apply it into your physical experience of your cycle – dress in the colours that resonate with you at that time of the month, wear your hair in the way that feels right for that archetype. Move in the way that you associate with that archetype. Create an animal totem for each of the archetypes...

Materials

First you need to choose the art materials that you wish to work with – something which allows quick work is better, as this is responsive, intuitive work – so if you choose paints, then acrylics, gouache or water colour, not oils. Clay feels lovely between the fingers for a very tactile, sensual experience. Pastels (chalky ones, not oil pastels) are great for beginning creatives as they are soft and forgiving, you can cover a lot of space quickly with them and if you are unhappy with something you can rub it out with your finger.

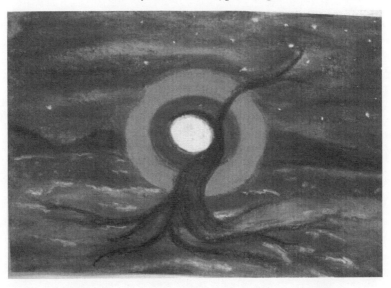

Set up your space

Make it somewhere where you can work undisturbed. Or if you are working alongside your children (as I often do) make it clear that you are working on your special project and they are working on theirs. Ensure that they are settled with their work before you begin.

Have all the materials you will need to hand and make sure surfaces are protected. Switch off your phone. You may want to light incense or smudge the space with sage. Perhaps have some music on which feels sacred to you – choose it according to the energy you are working with – enchantress music would be very different to mother music!

Centre yourself

Before you start your work, centre yourself with a few deep, mindful breaths. Place your hands on your belly, breathe in and out, bringing your attention to your womb. Bring your attention to where in your cycle you are. Have to hand the Integrated Menstrual Chart on page 37 of this book as a reference.

Visualisation

Concentrate on the archetype and answer the following questions instinctively, without excessive rationalisation and logical thought. There are no right or wrong answers, this is your interpretation. You can jot down your ideas if it helps:

o What colours do you associate with this archetype?

o What natural forms?

o What objects?

o What physical posture?

o What energy levels?

o What symbols?

o Where does she live?

o With whom?

o How does she wear her hair?

o What clothes does she wear?

o How does she move?

o What animal might she be?

o What element do you associate with her?

Exercise one – full series

In this exercise you will create a series of four pictures, each worked quickly and intuitively to express the archetypes. You will need four pieces of paper, one for each archetype.

Pick a colour for the virgin and start working, holding the key words which resonate with you about her in your mind as you work, keeping in mind the season, her element etc.

Then after ten minutes move onto the mother. After another ten minutes move on to the enchantress and finally the wise woman.

Step back and behold them, now you have the series, see if there is anything that you want to highlight about their similarities or differences. In this way you will produce a series of pictures in less than an hour.

Exercise two – cycle project

You can also work more deeply, throughout the course of a cycle. For this variation you commit to one hour (roughly) at each phase in your cycle. Still yourself and tune into the energy that is coursing around your body at that moment. Really feel it. And then take that onto the paper. Paint or draw yourself in this phase – what colours best express your mood, are you dynamic or still – what posture feels right to you?

Exercise three – branching out

Another time, perhaps you will choose to drum, dance, write monologues or poems, make a quilt or puppet, a piece of jewellery, or a self-portrait photograph for each different phase of your cycle.

Giving expression to these energies is fulfilling and insightful and can only lead you to greater self-knowledge.

If you are a professional artist, it might also lead you into some deep, personal works which profoundly touch the women who see them.

3

CHARTING YOUR CYCLE

Often we can feel overwhelmed and confused by the seeming turbulence of our bodies and unpredictability of our moods. I thoroughly recommend charting for a few months, to get a deep understanding of how your body and moods change throughout your cycle.

There are many ways to keep track of your cycle:

o   marking the expected date of your period in your diary

o   charting symptoms for Fertility Awareness – to aid conception or contraception

o   charting symptoms in a journal for healing PMT

o   keeping a moon diary – where you chart your symptoms alongside the moon's phases

o   using a moon dial

o   with a moon bracelet

(For stockists of all of these see the Resources section.)

I have been charting my cycle for many years, in different ways:

o   scientifically as a natural contraceptive method, noting the changes in discharge and body temperature. (NB: this produced two surprise babies for us!)

o   to give me insight in to my PMT noting what foods, events and parts of my cycle were in need of attention and healing

o   directly into my daily diary, both with moon cycles and without, to see what impact and correlation the moon has on my cycles

o   and sometimes in more prosaic, descriptive form (see below).

Each method provides useful insight into your changing, cyclical self, by recording the tiny details which we usually notice, then forget or dismiss. Charting shows us physiological and emotional patterns over the course of the month, and makes us more mindful of our eating, self-care regime, energy levels and fertility.

OOO

A cycle

As a way of illustrating the dynamic journey of the menstrual cycle, what better way than to share with you one of my own cycles? In this narrative you might recognise yourself and your own patterns which previously had gone unnoticed. (NB In talking about cycles, day one is the first day of bleeding.)

Day one
For the past couple of days I have known that my moon time is approaching. I know from the sky: the moon has gone and the nights are really dark. I know because as I was putting the children to bed, I wanted them to hurry up and be gone. I found their chirping voices too high energy, too much. I needed the smooth, slow darkness of my own mind. I wanted to be alone with my thoughts, to sink into them like a warm bath. Once they were in bed I felt drawn to my tarot cards and my journal.

Before I would have ignored these subtle signals until they were blaring and I was losing my temper. But last night I just stated quietly that I was coming near the end of my patience and energy and needed to be alone.

Day two
A surge of energy. If I am not careful I jump on board and quickly overdo it. It doesn't take much to make me exhausted – rather like during pregnancy, you have to learn to pace yourself, and I am a very slow learner. This time I organise an impromptu party. And then wish I hadn't! For two days afterwards I am pretty much bed-ridden with exhaustion.

Days three and four
I feel fat and blobby. I hate my clothes and my body. I just want to be left alone. Please, please everyone go away and leave me be! I lie or sit all the time. Chocolate is my friend, though I try not to eat too much. My work, which has been flying, seems to lose its focus and direction. I feel at sea, as though I have nothing in the world to say or give. I just need to be quiet and alone.

Day five
With my bleeding gone I feel the need to purify, to cleanse. I always have a sacred bath at this point, a literal washing away of the smell and feel of menstruation. It is a time for sloughing off dead skin and old feelings, to break fresh and clean into the new cycle. I don't like having baths during my moon time so it always feels like a real treat to have one. I luxuriate with a rose candle, bubble bath and steam rising up.

Days six to eight
My libido starts to rise. I feel buzzy and alive downstairs. My heart energy rises, I want to be close and affectionate, where only three days ago I desired nothing more than to be alone and untouched.

Days nine to twelve
My energy is soaring. With the clear flow of my ovulatory phase I celebrate with my sexual being. This is the fertile time, when all my children were conceived. It is a time for creativity – with body and soul. I have so many projects that I want to start right now!

Days thirteen and fourteen

Full moon is here and with it my ovulation – I feel deeply connected to the openness of the moon. I also feel a little crampy at this time of the month. I head outside and dance in the moonlight, and give thanks for all I have.

Days fifteen to nineteen

My energy feels clear and flowing, I am focused and creative and have huge amounts of energy – I could take over the world right now! I enjoy nourishing myself and my family, and entertaining friends. I fill my fridge and freezer with meals to sustain us when I no longer feel like cooking.

Days twenty to twenty four

I notice my energy levels starting to lessen – I am between the worlds, neither ovulatory nor pre-menstrual.

Days twenty five to twenty seven

A tireder, heavier energy emerges, I feel sluggish, and everything is an effort. I would really just like to curl up like a cat in a cosy chair in front of a roaring fire, and not be bothered. I bawl in front of a soppy TV program and growl about my husband's imperfections. I snap impatiently at the kids in the morning rush, then burst into tears.

Day twenty eight

I need to be nurtured, and I know I don't want a bath. I get this sense of not wanting to be in water just approaching my period. I need warming food, a blanket round my shoulders, to curl up in a seat and soak up gentle goodness. I put on a nourishing women's summit broadcast and soak in gentle feminine wisdom. And chocolate, of course chocolate! My absolute **need** for chocolate reaches a crescendo in the week before my period. It is so strong. And so necessary: dark, comforting warmth that soothes me.

I have also noticed that in the few hours before my period I suddenly become sexually alert and responsive, just as I do at ovulation. And then these feelings totally disappear for the next five days. I am not a sex during my period gal. No way, siree! This is my retreat time. It is a time for woolly socks, cosy jumpers, crying at girly films, and did I mention chocolate?

And you...

How much of this sounds familiar to you from your own cycle?

And where does your cycle differ?

Have you charted before? Which aspects worked, and which didn't?

What kind of charting calls to you?

What do you want to understand more about? PMT, fertility, your moods?

Why not start a moon diary? Each day of your cycle note down a couple of words about your emotional state, energy levels and any physical symptoms to begin to see the course of your moon journey which your hormones and body are following.

Using a moon dial

A moon dial gives a great reminder of the repetitive, cyclical nature of your menstrual cycle and is particularly helpful for visual learners. The moon dial can be an interactive journey of discovery of oneself in relation to the moon's own cycles. Through exploring and aligning theses cycles we can create liberation, by balancing our whole being.

With your moon dial you can:

o   note the phase of the moon relative to your cycle

o   place the date next to each day to keep track easily

o   note physical symptoms, general health, energy levels, activity and dreams.

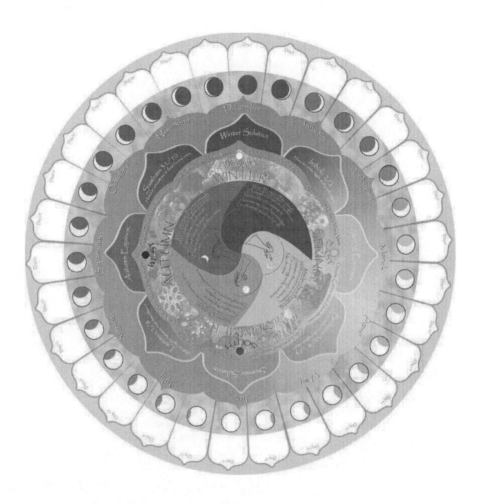

Moon dial mandala created by Zoe Shekinah. Available to buy from
www.earthlightcollective.com and www.thehappywomb.com

Charting by the sky

Having used many different methods, I have become exquisitely aware of the minor changes in my body: my mood, my cravings, my emotions and my needs. Though I no longer chart my cycle on paper, or use calendar dates, I always know where I am both within my own individual cycle (because of my physical and emotional self-awareness) and because it is directly aligned to the moon's cycles, within nature's larger cycles too.

I enjoy charting by the sky, rather than on a calendar, which is, after all sun-based, not moon-based. If I use the calendar on the wall, my cycle does not fall on the same day of the month; it always feels slightly "off kilter". I found that noting it in my diary meant that it stood, looming over me, that ominous, foreboding date of "I'm getting my period" so I can't go swimming/ see friends etc. It became a negative, dreaded thing. It was also a date set in stone so that I was either early or late perhaps by a day, or a few hours. And then I would panic that I was pregnant if it was late – cue multiple unneeded pregnancy tests. All this set me up for self-judgement and dread, not self-acceptance and love.

Now I know that around full moon time I ovulate and get a rush of energy, virility and fertility, just as the moon is reaching her full power. I moon dance, celebrate with other women, and have wonderful couple time with my husband. On the dark moon, I begin to bleed. And so with a general awareness of the skies I know where I am at in relation to where the moon is on her journey.

If you told me I would feel or believe this even five years ago I would have laughed at you. That is why I say, take this book where you are on your own journey. Some of it might be relevant now. Other bits might be stashed in the "for later" memory file. And some might never be your thing.

Know where you are on your journey and all will be well.

4

PUTTING THE MOON BACK INTO MENSTRUATION

A growing understanding of ecology and feedback systems has led us to see that every living organism is in constant contact with its surrounding environment and continuously influenced by it.

We tend to think that our biological rhythms are independent of the environment, but many of them were originally acquired through interaction with the outside world. It is not by chance that women's menstrual cycles and the moon's phase correspond, any more than it is coincidence that all people have built in diurnal rhythms of approximately the same length. At one time moonlight and sunlight actually controlled such functions directly but through evolution these rhythms have become incorporated into our biological systems.

Prof. Kerstin Uvnas Moberg, *The Oxytocin Factor: Tapping the Hormone of Calm, Love and Healing*

Moon Time

A cycle is the basic unit of life: birth, growth, transformation, decline and death, followed once again by birth. This process of expansion and contraction, activity and rest can be seen in every life form on the planet, in the seasons and the phases of the moon.

Our bodies are in constant, rhythmic change, but because so much of this is happening beneath our waking consciousness, we can feel out of control, or "all at sea". When we begin to notice the pattern of these cycles, their repetitive nature, their connection to nature beyond us, we can begin to feel not victims unprepared for the weather, but sailors, prepared by attending to the storm warnings, the pull of the tides, and the placing of the stars and moon for navigation.

The most common menstrual pattern is to bleed on the dark moon and to ovulate at full moon. That the 28 day menstrual cycle correlates with the moon's cycle, as well as the fact that women living in close proximity cycle together, are some of the mysterious elements of the menstrual cycle which science and the world at large seem to have little interest in. But once women are aware of this, it adds an extra dimension to their appreciation of the intricate sensitivities of their bodies to the natural world around them. It is truly remarkable that the pull of a distant astronomical body has such an impact on our own small selves.

Before the advent of electric light in the late nineteenth century, women's ovulation was primarily activated by their hormonal response to the brightness of the full moon at night. In our modern era however, street lighting, electric lights inside, artificial hormones, pollutants and stress have contributed to women's cycles being more staggered throughout the month, with some bleeding rather than ovulating at full moon (known as the red moon cycle) , and many others unconnected to the moon's cycles at all. Women who have charted their cycles and experienced menstruation at dark and full moon report feeling more "in flow" and "attuned to themselves" when they bleed on the dark moon.

We are not the only species influenced by the moon – corals spawn, wolves howl, most mammals go into labour and turtles lay eggs at the full moon. Traditionally farmers planted and harvested by the moon's cycles as well.

Putting the Moon Back into Menstruation

There is increasing evidence from research on people and animals alike, that the destruction of biological rhythms has implications for an organism's health and general well-being. Our bodies were born on this Earth, programmed by our genes and enculturation to be tied to the sun's daily rhythms for waking and sleeping, and the moon for our menstrual cycles.

Scientists show that our physical growth happens at night. New mothers and babies require much higher levels of sleep and rest. And so do menstruating women. For thousands of years farmers have known about the importance of allowing fields to lie fallow to re-balance their nutrients and growing potential.

It is just the same with us women. As life givers we are given the clues in the form of PMT that in order to be healthy, bring forth new life and create new work and nurture others, it is essential that we rest and regenerate.

We live in a culture which demands that we are "turned on" all the time. Always bright and happy. Always available for intercourse – both sexual and otherwise with people. Psychologist Peter Suedfeld observes that we are all "chronically stimulated, socially and physically and are probably operating as a simulation level higher than that for which our species evolved."

It is up to us to value rest and fallow time. We must demand it for ourselves to ensure our health.

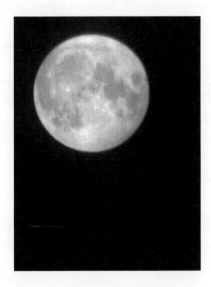

Celebrating full moon

Cultures around the world celebrate the full moon and its vibrant energies in different ways – from full moon parties on Thai beaches to Jewish family feasts.

Spending time out in the bright light of the full moon is a magical experience, even for the most cynical of us. If you are looking to re-align your menstrual cycle with the moon's cycle, exposure to the full moon light can have a very powerful effect.

For those of you who enjoy deepening their physical connection to the moon, here are some of my favourite energising full moon activities.

Moon dancing

There are full moon circles that gather to celebrate the full moon. Often for women only, they moon dance – fully clothed or naked – to music, drums or in silence, in groups or alone. Each month is often given a theme to focus the participants' intentions.

According to a co-ordinator, Becky, *"We can get extra magical benefits of our moon circle connection – healing and love light. Make a list of all the things you are grateful for, either written down or across your heart. The moon energy combined with your presence and awareness will infuse your body, mind and spirit –like a thankful tea, steeped full of love, moonlight, and thankfulness that you can drink for the next month."*

Women communicate on-line via many of the Facebook groups and blogs listed in the Resources section. In this way, we create a virtual community of moon sisters, connecting the dancing dots all over the planet, and call to mind the other women who are joining us, knowing where in the world they are.

Moon bathing

Go outside and feel the electric glow of moonlight and chill on your skin, take your shoes off, perhaps even your top in mid-summer! Feel the dew beneath your feet, perhaps wash your face in it. Imagine this purifying your body-mind.

Invoke the timeless wisdom of the moon into your body and soul. Sing or chant, whisper your prayers. Root yourself in the earth, feel your sensitivities rise, your awareness grow, of your body, of the earth beneath your feet and the heavens above you, and your own place in this magical plane.

Put a blanket on the grass if it is damp and lie on your back, looking up at the moon, the stars and the vast expanse of the heavens.

Celebrate the full moon and the rise in your fertility and desire with your partner – or alone: dance together, make love, have a moonlight picnic and frolic in the dew.

Enjoy a sensual moonlight swim or moonlight stroll.

Open your curtains and sleep in the bright moon light.

Or even, just as you walk through your house, turning off your lights before you go to bed, take a moment to gaze up at the moon through your window, and allow yourself to breathe and be fully present.

5

FINDING OUR VOICES

Often as women we are silenced – especially when it comes to our bodies. What we said has been considered irrelevant or just plain wrong. We might have had things to say which upset people, or made them uncomfortable. And so we learnt to silence ourselves.

I strongly believe that a large amount of the anger and tearfulness we experience pre-menstrually, is our body's way of expressing the deep truths which we try to stifle.

In allowing us to off-load toxic thoughts and feelings, in forcing us to make uncomfortable changes in our unhealthy lives, our female bodies are pushing us towards greater health and happiness. It just doesn't feel that way at the time!

The American midwife extraordinaire, Ina May Gaskin, notes in her book *Spiritual Midwifery*, how women's throat and uterine sphincters are closely related when giving birth. If a mother can release and open one, by speaking her truth, chanting or singing then the other also releases and relaxes as if by magic, and the birth can progress. So to continue that thought, if we can release our fertile, creative flow through our voice, then we find ease with our bleeding time.

For hundreds of years women have been silenced so as not to bring shame or negative attention upon their husband or family. A woman should only talk about nice subjects of good taste, and certainly not anger people. She was taught how to walk and talk to be pleasing to the eye and ear. Her voice should be light and breezy. Her art, should she be allowed to make it, should be beautiful. Her appetites have been suppressed, her passions seen as suspect. Her flesh too was moulded into tight corsets or skinny jeans as fashion dictated. We have been denied being ourselves, with our voices, in our bodies, with our thoughts.

And you...

What is it that you would really like to say? And to whom?

Create a safe space and allow yourself to speak your truth – without needing to justify or explain, simply hear your voice speaking your full truth. Every last bit of it. Ungag yourself. Free your voice. Give yourself permission to let your feelings be as they are. Speak your truth – and own it.

o   You can do this by journaling. Putting your seething, unexpressed, and seemingly inexpressible, taboo feelings into words is a massive step in healing, letting go and finding clarity for yourself.

o   But even more powerful is speaking out loud. So if nothing else, read aloud what you have written in the privacy of your own room or moon lodge.

o   More powerful still is to be heard by someone else (usually **not** the person it is directed at, at this point. The purpose of this is to purge your powerful feelings uncensored.) Ensure absolute confidentiality – perhaps a counsellor or therapist, your women's group, red tent, a close friend or partner.

o   Or post on an anonymous blog. **The Honesty Conspiracy** (**www.honestyconspiracy.blogspot.com**) is one such blog devoted to women's healing. Anyone can contribute in complete anonymity to voice their truth and receive support and feedback.

o   After this venting and release, after reflection and possible feedback, then you can clarify what, and if you do want to communicate to the person involved, or what action you need to take. Then you can act with conviction and speak in a way that your message can be heard. At other times, simply allowing yourself to hear and express your truth is all that is needed to find peace and healing and to move forward.

OOO

The naming of parts

The first stage of acceptance, self-love and healing of our bodies is to lighten up about them. Many of us were brought up without appropriate or comfortable words for our female genitalia. They were shrouded in silence and mystery, and not to be talked about.

Let's break the silence on our bodies together. Let's get creative and re-claim the language we use to talk about them for ourselves. Let's create a shared language of words that we feel comfortable with.

There is a Second World War poem called The Naming of Parts by Henry Reed, which I remember studying at school. Written in steady rhyming verse, it deals with guns, death, war and speaking the unspeakable.

But this is a women's book. So here is my own Naming of Parts – free flowing and feminine!

The naming of parts:

a thought poem on what we call ourselves

Without words we have no meaning.

Without words we have no reality.

We have only silence.

And shame.

Here is our naming of parts.

I have never liked **menstruation** as a word.

Why should my woman's time have "men" in it?

And as for **menses** – NO! It sounds like faeces.

I was lucky not to be brought up with "**the curse**", though many were.

And **period** just feels empty, final ... period!

There is no image, nothing to attach to.

Our language shapes our perception.

Some have kindly women:

Aunt Flo and **Grandmother Moon**...

I choose words that work for me.

Moon Time

Moon time...

I envisage the egg, a perfect white globe, full and blooming at ovulation, sailing down a red river.

This is my moon time, a time when I feel moon-faced and blank.

The moon is an image of beauty and light.

And **blood time**.

This is what I call it for my children – flesh of my flesh –

"Mummy's blood time"...

It does – as they say – exactly what it says on the tin!

Bleeding does not feel so good for me.

Bleeding implies endless, gushing, active, illness, distress...

Which doesn't exactly make my heart leap!

And now, other pressing matters, needing names...

Many of us do not have a comfortable word for "**down there**".

For many becoming mother to a little girl forces us to have a name...

For me **vagina** is too clinical,

And anyway, then you need the addendum of **vulva** –

Vulva is creepy, slithering, a snake...

My father called it a **pussy** – but it is no cat!

And **fanny** – yuck!

There's a reason the American reserve that word for the back bum.

Finding Our Voices

Which leads us neatly onto...

Front bum – uh-uh – no shit comes out of here!

But you know what I like?

I like **lady garden**, (though I wouldn't say it out loud!)

It is exotic, beautiful, night scented and balmy, with dark corners for romantic trysts and roses in full bloom.

In reality I say **bits**, or **down there** or **"there"**

It always helps to point!

Yup, liberated is my middle name!

To our daughters we call it a **yoni**.

And I'm working on mine being one too!

I like that word a lot.

Yoni means **sacred space** in Sanskrit – **origin, source** – it refers to the entire genital system

And that feels good, to have a complete term.

It's holistic!

In India there are **altars dedicated to the Yoni**,

Whole temples decorated with them!

Imagine!

This is good and right, I think.

"Blessed is the yoni through which we all came to be."

Our friends say yoni too.

Though the kids at school wouldn't know what a yoni was if it hit them in the face...

Which might not be a great idea!

Though by the time it hit them in the face, they'd know!

What is yours?

Whisper it quietly, I won't tell a soul!

And then we have the **inner sanctum,**

A clinical **uterus**

Or a warm, embracing **womb.**

The magic cave as I call it with my children.

The place where I once cradled their growing beings within me.

And the **cervix** – sometimes pinched closed like a child that won't take their medicine

Or an old lady who disapproves.

At times it feels like the tip of your nose.

Mine can **roar like a lion** at ten centimetres dilated.

I sang it open as I birthed my babes through its **portal**.

This truly is the **mouth of my womb** and of my woman soul.

I am woman – hear me roar!

I am woman – hear me moan!

I am woman!

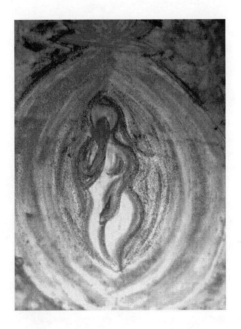

And you...

What do you call female body parts?

Do you like what you call them?

Is there another word or phrase that would work better for you?

How can you own it? How can you speak of it as yours, an unashamed part of you? Imagine if you could say its name as easily as saying "belly button" or "elbow".

Give it as much thought as you would naming your first born child. Make sure you have a name which runs well off the tongue. Do you need to use a different name for your partner and your doctor?

What name makes your heart lift rather than bows your head with shame?

If you have children, what do you call female parts with them?

How comfortable do you feel with this?

Is it easier naming male genitals than female in public?

And now

I offer you a sacred invitation:

To take a moment to lighten up about your female parts.

How could you interact creatively with your female parts? How could you get more comfortable with what you physically are? How can you get your mind, around your body?

Perhaps you could...

o   Have an official naming ceremony for your woman's body. With one VIP guest – YOU!

o   Visualise your ovaries ovulating.

o   Meditate on your womb.

o   Draw your yoni... or make a print with it!

o   Dance your womb contractions in labour.

o   Sing or chant your period pain.

o Moan your orgasms loud.

o Paint your belly with henna.

What comes up for you as you consider doing any of these things? Do they freak you out? Revolt you? Scare you? Make you laugh out loud or shrivel up inside?

Do you dare? If so, watch what comes up whilst you are doing any of these acts.

This is the wall of silence and taboo that you are breaking. How strong an influence is it in your life, your choices, your behaviour, even in private? This is what we are working with (or against!) This level of resistance is what stands between you and finding peace and belonging in your body. Baby step by baby step we are finding acceptance of what we are made frim, and who we are.

Feel the fear and do it anyway!

OOO

New stories

Along with new language for our bodies which empowers us, we also need new frameworks for understanding ourselves. We need new stories, new creation myths. We can create them anew, or we can trawl back through our culture and others to reclaim our stories of what it means to be a woman. Stories have power. Let us learn new stories that we can tell to our daughters, that we can use for ourselves.

Those of us growing up in the Judaeo-Christian tradition had the myth of Adam and Eve as our Creation story. In this the Creator God tells Eve that because of her disobedience she will be made to suffer in her childbearing. Our menstruation is part of our childbearing cycle, and therefore our suffering is seen as both natural, and deserved divine punishment, for our female transgressions.

Other cultures and other times have had different understandings of the female body and its innate rhythms and wisdom that they transmitted to their women. Other cultures have honoured the menstrual blood as wise. Other cultures have honoured their women for their life-giving abilities.

And our culture can too. But it starts from us. It starts from changing our own beliefs about what it means to be a woman, and the stories we tell, and believe, about ourselves.

In expanding our knowledge and understanding of other stories and cultures, we come to see that many of the beliefs that we hold, about our bodies and selves, that we have previously accepted as truths are nothing more than cultural dogma. In seeing this, we can begin to remake our own belief systems according to our own unique physical and soul-level experiences.

If you are interested in the power of myth and story in the creation of our identities, may I draw your attention to Clarissa Pinkola Estes' seminal book on the subject, *Women Who Run With The Wolves*. She has a number of powerful retellings of fairy stories including "Little Red Shoes" and "Seal Skin, Soul Skin" which impart profound soul truths about how to be a cycling woman in the world, how to honour our wildness, our blood mysteries and our need to retreat.

The following story is one from the Native American tradition, retold by one of their elders, Nicholas Noblewolf. It tells of their understanding of the significance of a woman's moon time and how it should be respected by herself, the menfolk and the tribe.

OOO

A moon time myth

As told by Nicholas Noble Wolf

A long time ago, women did as they do now—they held the family, they held the power (life-force) for the family, they held the happiness and joy, they held the sorrow and disappointments. After time, the negative emotions and heartache that the women took upon themselves on behalf of their families would begin to weigh them down. The women would become sick and finally, could no longer take on the burdens of the family. Yet the nature to do so had been imbued into them by Creator.

One day, a woman was out in the forest, crying because the burden had become so great, when Raven heard her and asked, "Mother, why do you cry?"

The woman responded, "I love my family so very much. I hold my family in my heart and soul, but the pains of life have filled me up. I can no longer help my family. I can no longer take their burdens from them. I just don't know what to do."

Raven responded, "I understand the pain you feel, as I feel it also. I will go and ask Grandmother Ocean if she knows what to do." So Raven flew to the ocean and shared with Grandmother the plight of the women.

Grandmother Ocean responded, "If the women will come to me, I will wash their pain from them, but this won't help the ones who are far away. Let me ask my sister, Grandmother Moon, if she can help."

So Grandmother Ocean spoke to her sister of the women's plight. Grandmother Moon responded, "I am the power of the feminine. I will send into the women, my sisters, your waters carrying my power. Once every moon cycle, you shall come into the women through me and purify them." And, she did this. So ever since then, every woman has a time each moon cycle when she embodies the power of the moon and flows the cleansing of the ocean. We call this the woman's time of the moon, or moon-time.

Moon Time

It is each woman's responsibility to take the time when she is in her time of the moon to purify. It is the responsibility of the men to give the women the opportunity to do so.

Nicholas Noble Wolf

This story was taken from an article first published in Sacred Hoop magazine 2000. It is republished here with the author's permission.

www.nicholasnoblewolf.com

6

MOURNING MOON

It's all very well to talk about welcoming your moon time. But what if the splash of red is the last thing you wanted to see?

o Perhaps you are trying, and struggling to get pregnant, and the appearance of your period feels like confirmation of another failure.

o Perhaps your period means another round of expensive and exhausting IVF has failed.

o Perhaps you are a few days late or even a few weeks and you have mixed feelings about it.

o Perhaps you are hoping that you are pregnant, or know that you are. This is not just a period, this is a miscarriage, and with it might come heartbreak, soul wrenching loss.

o Perhaps it is a reminder of an abortion – wanted or unwanted.

It is more important than ever at these times to follow the private moon lodge/self-care process, which we shall cover later.

Techniques for dealing with loss

Get your feelings out, see them on the page, hear them out loud for what they are. Allow yourself time and space to grieve, to mourn, to wail. Moon time is a natural time of loss. Ride its wave, allow its dark energy to take your sadness and pain in its flow. Allow your body to scream out its sadness and frustration. It is normal and natural and OK.

o   Journal your feelings.

o   Share them with other women – perhaps in person with a special friend, sister or mother.

o   Or perhaps by email or letter.

o   Phone a support line.

o   Talk to your health care practitioner or counsellor.

o   Beat a pillow. Or lie on your bed and thrash your arms and legs.

o   Sing, stamp, wail, dance, scream – move and vocalise however you can.

o   Dissolve into the sadness.

o   Allow yourself to be held, to be rocked and cradled like a baby and comforted.

o   Allow someone to brush your hair, to stroke your hand, to rub your shoulders. Feel that love and care and expect nothing more from yourself than to be a conduit of your feelings.

o   Take time to do a healing meditation.

o   Wear a poppy for remembrance.

o   Keep mementoes – photographs, drawings, a symbol, the remains, close to you – in a locket, your handbag or on your dressing table.

o   Have a place in nature – the ocean, a special tree, a mountain – to go to when you feel bereft.

o   Pick or buy yourself some flowers, make a garland or wreath.

o   Bury or burn something in the ground.

It is real. It is allowed. It is not the end of everything.

Even though it might feel like it.

If your loss was a while ago, do not be surprised if these feeling re-emerge with every moon time. Take the opportunity each time to work through them more deeply, to heal yourself a little more, so that you might free yourself from being bound to them.

Allowing as the blood flows that your tears flow too. Allow yourself to empty, to shed a skin, to feel the darkness and be in that place. And then, as your body begins its journey to ripeness and fertility once more, allow yourself to follow your body's lead back into the light, embracing life in its fullness and renewed possibilities.

7

PMT BUSTERS

Our menstrual cycle is our barometer of our being.

Jane Hardwicke Collings, shamanic midwife

PMT (pre-menstrual tension) or PMS (pre-menstrual syndrome) can include any (or all) of the following symptoms:

o   abdominal bloating and water retention

o   tearfulness

o   being snappy, angry, short-tempered, impatient

o   cramping

o   lower back ache

o   dizziness, nausea, fainting

o   migraine or headaches

o   forgetfulness, brain fog or difficulty making decisions

o spots, greasy skin and hair

o tender, lumpy, larger breasts

For some women these symptoms may start over a week before their period comes and may continue throughout their bleeding time. This is no small matter if two weeks out of every month are filled with physical and emotional suffering.

In this chapter I share a number of useful natural solutions for PMT. If you need something more specially tailored for you, find someone who takes you seriously and whom you trust. Many women find that conventional doctors can be very dismissive of PMT symptoms – having the attitude: "it's just part of being female, so stop complaining!" And many may seek to cure you of your problems by prescribing the Pill. I remember that my doctor when I was a teen told me I'd have to learn to live with it and it would get better after I had children – what a great help that was!

If you are tempted to take the Pill to alleviate PMT symptoms, or your young daughter has this suggested to her, be sure to read the book *The Pill: Are you sure it's for you?* (reviewed in Chapter 10) before doing so, to ensure that you are fully informed about it.

Somewhat incredibly, especially if you suffer badly from PMT, many menstrual researchers have discovered that PMT is a condition almost exclusively found in the Western world. Indeed, it is a complaint that women and medical professionals alike in other cultures have no comprehension of.

PMT has been attributed to a combination of: pollution, poor diets, raised stress levels, 24-7 lifestyles and the status of women in our culture. In the afterword to *The Wise Wound,* authors Penelope Shuttle and Peter Redgrove state: "Society apparently has amplified the menstrual taboo by creating a diet [and lifestyle] that is OK for men but which harms women's menstrual cycles."

It seems that we have built a culture which optimises PMT, depression and exhaustion, rather than women's health. It is time to start taking this back, one woman's life at a time.

The Crazy Woman

The emotional side of PMT is the raw, primal female voice unleashed, your primal power saying: enough – I need space, time, freedom and expression – let me out!

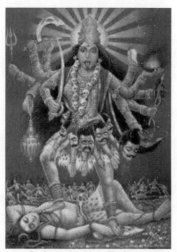

Indian Goddess Kali

This is the Crazy Woman. She was depicted and revered in ancient goddesses: Kali, Medea and Hecate, but our modern cultures have no place for her and no image of her. We fear her destructiveness inside ourselves and she is deeply threatening to our society.

We dare not admit to her for fear of being deemed "unable to cope", out of concern that our children might be taken from us or that we might be hospitalized in a mental institution. And so our Crazy Woman side is further denied, pushed away, or medicated with anti-depressants, self-harm, eating disorders or alcohol.

"Crazy Woman does not really wish to kill you. She wishes to maim your talents and paralyse your ability; she wishes to strip you of all your sacredness. She pulls your sanity and tests you, trying to pull you away from your centre." **Lynn V Andrews, Meta Arts magazine**

The Crazy Woman emerges for me after too much unbroken child-caring time, sleep deprivation or too little creative head space. I get cranky and snappy. If this is compounded over weeks and weeks I suffer from PMT, migraines and depression. The results aren't pretty. I want to see blood, make pain. I want to do damage, destroy everything which on a different day I hold dear. I want to smash plates, slam doors, hurt my children, scream at the top of my lungs, even kill myself. But I don't. So I shout, or drive the car a bit too fast, or stuff my face with unhealthy food. I want to run, to hide, to quit once and for all. I have had enough.

Denial of our creative selves, lack of space and time to be or reflect are lures for the Crazy Woman. She emerges, raging, crying, shouting, threatening, hands shaking, face pale. But rather than let her out, we try to shut her up and then blame everyone else for her enslavement and our feeling of being trapped.

When you are tired and drained and you have given every drop of energy, love, patience. When you need a break, some head space, some body space and just can't get it. Then you feel truly like you are going crazy, like you are dying inside.

And this is right in a way – we are experiencing the psychic suffocation of our creative selves, when we are so subsumed by external demands, when we do not have time to tend our creative fires, to unleash our imaginative power, plumb our depths, to breathe consciously, to reflect, to play.

Honouring your Crazy Woman

How can we find safe expression for the Crazy Woman? How can we be true to her and ourselves? How can we find balance in our lives so that she need not emerge too often or destructively?

As crazy as it might sound, rather than push her away, we need to honour her.

So next time your Crazy Woman comes to visit, don't run and hide from her. Welcome her as an honoured guest.

Copy down her words in your journal and heed them well. Stop what you are doing and drink tea with her. Dance to her wild tune, play your drums with and shake your rattles. Take her to bed and ravish her with sleep, let her guide you into other realms of your consciousness. Trust her rather than refuse her. Let her lead you by the hand and thank her for her presence.

She is you. Your shadow side with lessons to teach you about what you choose to hide away. She calls your deepest soul attention to that which you refuse to shine your light on. She may terrify you, embarrass you, mess up your carefully made plans and your carefully done mascara, but she is your soul sister, your twin self. She has been scorned and rejected, demonised throughout history. Open your arms and your heart to her and her lessons. Welcome your soul sister back.

And you...

What have you learnt about the Crazy Woman – from your mother, grandmother, aunts, teachers, female friends? Was she acceptable or locked away, the mad woman in the attic? Was she papered over with niceness and face powder? Was she medicated with anti-depressants or alcohol? Did she emerge in screaming fits or suicide attempts?

Grab a sheet of paper and put down all the words you associate with her.

Take your journal and write down her last few visits – why did she come? What invited her into your life? How did she express herself? What did she want? What was her message?

And now that you have a tangible sense of her, how could you represent her or symbolise her? If you have an altar space in your house, put an image or reminder on it of her.

To listen to an audio presentation of Honouring Your Crazy Woman which I shared on Day 14 of The World's Biggest Summit visit www.worldsbiggestsummit.com.

It is also available on the resources section of my website www.thehappywomb.com

PMT and motherhood

What strikes me reading through a lot of the material on menstruation is that is seems oddly detached from the fruits of the menstrual cycle: children. In *The Wise Wound*, Penelope Shuttle notes that there is no research done on the impact of a mother's PMT on her children. Yet think what a massive impact this has on them. This is yet another area where we need to learn to break the silence and find new ways of living and mutual support.

I saw my mother struggle badly with PMT. She seemed to have it for two out of every four weeks. She was like a bear, and any tiny thing was an excuse for her to shout and scream and behave (in my eyes) unforgivably. It seemed to me to be a "get out of jail free card" for her moods and emotions: "it's not my fault, I've got PMT".

So we all suffered along with her. She was disempowered by her emotions. And we were disempowered by them too. It felt like the whole house was cowering from her and her bloody (excuse the pun!) period.

And so when my time came, and for years afterwards, I tried to hide mine underground, because I didn't want to be like her. I didn't want to make it everyone else's problem. But that is easier said than done. Especially, as I was to discover, when you have young children.

Perhaps children are not part of your plan now, or ever. But most women at some point in their moon life will have to balance the constant energetic requirements of children with their own changing energy cycles.

For me this has been an enormous learning curve, because at just the time when I am really starting to tune into my own rhythms, I have three children making demands of me – needing me to wake in the night to breastfeed or settle them, wanting me to play high energy games when all I want to do is lie on the sofa. I find it deeply challenging being able to feel my body's rhythm and know how best I can meet this, and yet be constantly prevented from doing this because of the needs of my children and their lack of understanding.

In other cultures and other times women would not be left to care for children alone, in isolation. Instead it was the job of the community to care for, feed and educate the young of the tribe, and women would share their mothering and household chores between them.

Bear this in mind during your moon time. Join together with friends, let your children play together as you cook a meal to share. Or exchange childcare so that you can both have a couple of hours to yourself.

OOO

Positively menstrual!

So how can we transform PMT? I have found that this simple four part process works wonders in my own life, especially in combatting martyr mentality:

o   Step one – Feel/ identify your needs

o   Step two – Claim your needs

o   Step three – Make it **your** problem, not everyone else's

o   Step four – Make your peace – express gratitude and seek forgiveness

As soon as you model how you can positively meet your needs, you will find those around you following your lead and helping to support this. Whereas if you are attacking them and they are having to be defensive, they are not going to feel very supportive or like giving you anything!

So let's re-name PMT:

Power of Moon Time.
Or
Positive Menstrual Time.

Learn to use your power wisely. Own it!

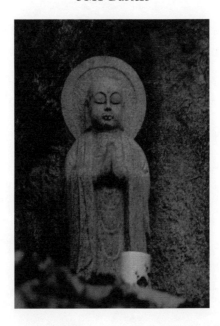

Instant PMT busters

Chances are if you have PMT right now you feel crappy and don't know where to start. You just want to feel better. Pick three of these and you'll be well on your way to feeling good. Can't choose? Just close your eyes, point to one. Then do it!

o In my grandmother's words: SIMPLIFY, SIMPLIFY, SIMPLIFY! This is your mantra for a better moon time.

o Relish your dream time. Ernest Hartmann, author of *The Biology of Dreaming*, has shown that our need for REM sleep increases in the pre-menstrual period and lack of it causes PMT.

o Ensure you have no major deadlines – either get work done early or renegotiate extra time for yourself so that days 28-3 are as clear of external obligation as they can be.

o Cook in advance for yourself and freeze the meals, go out to eat, get invited to others' houses, have your partner take over cooking duties, buy ready meals…

Moon Time

o Limit energetic or extended physical activity – no long walks or marathons!

o A short, gentle stroll outside does you the world of good to reconnect with yourself and nature and get the energy moving.

o Or perhaps a walking meditation

o Have you discovered womb yoga?

o Keep your clothing comfortable – especially if you get bloated or chilly at this time.

o Do something to make yourself look and feel beautiful – wear a special necklace, a lovely scent, a pretty scarf…

o Make no major decisions. Just don't do it to yourself!

o Take time every day for yourself.

o Create your own personal moon lodge – minimum half an hour devoted retreat and self-care.

o Try to get to bed in good time – late night stints will be with you soon enough.

o Get as much support you can for any big projects, especially events outside of your control – work events, Christmas, relatives visiting...

o Take the pressure off yourself with extra support where you need it in your life.

o Be open with those that you are close to that this is a time where you need to be gentle with yourself.

o Do everything you can to make yourself feel cherished NOT a patient or a victim – your mental attitude matters hugely.

o Scream into a pillow.

o Take ten conscious breaths.

PMT Busters

o Have a girly lunch with a friend.

o Let your hair down, your tears out and your feelings be heard.

o Write in your journal.

o Get a punch bag and beat it!

o Have an orgasm – they're great for releasing tensions in the yoni, and they give you a rush of serotonin and oxytocin to boost your mood.

o Choose one relationship issue to take action on. Do not try to change your world or those around you just because you are angry and frustrated. Just one clear communication, made in calmness of a need that you have and how you would like it to be met. Next month you get a chance to voice another.

o Bathe yourself in the positivity of others if you are feeling dark – uplifting books, films, blogs…

o Listen to something that lifts you – music, an inspirational speaker, birdsong…

o Tend your altar – add an image of the Crazy Woman.

o Do some receiving from your family: get a full body massage, a shoulder rub, a hug, a meal made for you…

o Snuggle up with a hot water bottle or castor oil pack.

o Brew up a pot of herbal tea.

o Go to the health food store and get some supplements for yourself.

o Eat chocolate!

o Recharge yourself with a pedicure, acupuncture, cranio-sacral therapy, reiki, chiropractic treatment…

o Start a dream journal – note down everything that comes through from your other layers of consciousness at this time.

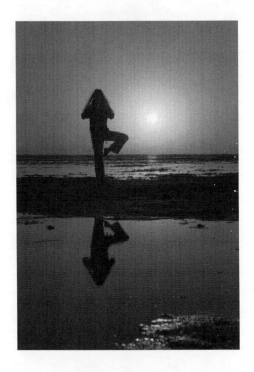

There is no shame in tears.
There is a need for anger.
Blood will flow.
Let yourself rest.
Speak your truth.
Follow your intuition.
Nurture your body.

8

NUTRITIONAL & HERBAL HEALING

We can do all the emotional healing in the world, but if we are not nurturing and nourishing our physical bodies we will never find good health. What we eat can impact our moods, create allergic responses and affect our energy levels. Part of our healing journey is becoming aware of how we respond to different foods at different times in our cycle.

Herbs are part of the traditional wise woman approach to health. Cultures around the world use the healing powers of plants to help support the female system from Chinese herbs (often given alongside acupuncture), to Ayurveda (alongside Yoga), Native American and traditional European wise woman herbalism. They have been used to promote fertility, abort unwanted foetuses, support breastfeeding, tone the uterus in preparation for birth and to lighten or induce bleeding.

Herbs tend to be much gentler than pharmaceuticals and work with the body, rather than simply repressing symptoms. They tend to have few, if any, unwanted side effects. However, they are still powerful external forces in the body and we need to have respect for herbs, in just the same way as we do for pharmaceutical medicines.

Herbs can be taken in capsules, teas or tinctures. They can be grown yourself, sourced from a health shop or herbalist.

If you are new to herbs I strongly recommend consulting with a herbalist or naturopath to help to focus and support your healing. If you have used herbs before, then be sure to consult a good herbal book or knowledgeable health food shop assistant to check of any contraindications for other medication you may be taking, breastfeeding implications and previous health complaints.

Below is a resource of herbal and nutritional remedies for easing moon time symptoms, and helping you to work with your cycles.

Please note I am not a trained herbalist. The list of herbs below is simply meant as information, not a prescription. Whilst I have sourced these suggestions from a range of reliable sources and I have tried many of them myself, I request that you seek further advice before taking them.

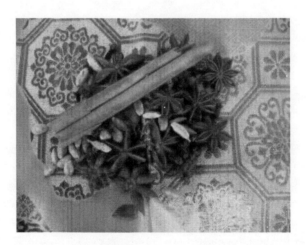

Supplements

o **Shatavari** – the Queen of Herbs for women. Its name means "she who has a hundred husbands" in Sanskrit. It is used in Ayurveda to enhance the libido, energise, lighten menstrual bleeding and generally support the female hormonal system.

o **St John's Wort** – for depressive symptoms. Because of regulations this is becoming increasingly difficult to source in the EU.

- o **Feverfew** – for migraine and headaches (can be eaten fresh in salads and sandwiches).

- o **Evening Primrose** – great for relieving PMS symptoms, taken ten days before bleeding starts – especially effective for easing tender breasts.

- o **Maca** – a Peruvian root, great for energy boosting, many add it to green smoothies along with **spirulina** for an instant nutritional hit.

- o **Quiet Life** – a natural supplement combining passiflora, lettuce, hops and valerian to calm anxiety and help natural sleep.

Teas

These can be bought loose, harvested from your garden, or bought as tea bags:

- o **Lemon Balm (Melissa)** – to soothe and relax.

- o **Red Raspberry Leaf** - tones the uterus and aids nausea.

- o **Nettle** - for iron. Tones the uterus, supports production of breast-milk and vitamin K.

- o **Cramp Bark** - for easing cramps!

- o **Motherwort** – good for cramping during menstruation and easing labour contractions and after-pains.

- o **Chamomile** to soothe, relax and help sleep.

- o **Shepherd's Purse** – to ease excessively heavy bleeding.

Herbal recipes

You can use tinctures in water or brew herbs together to make tea.

In *Thirteen Moons,* a herbalist suggests:

o A combination of red raspberry, cramp bark, squaw vine and black cohosh for general PMS symptoms.

Neal's Yard recommends:

o Motherwort, passiflora and skullcap for easing stress.

o Agnus castus and false unicorn for stabilising the hormones.

o Motherwort, chamomile, cramp bark, passiflora and raspberry to ease period pains.

o Dandelion and parsley leaves for relieving bloating.

My personal favourites...

o Rose-hip and hibiscus – red tea perfect for bleeding time ceremonies, and good source of vitamin C.

o Cinnamon, ginger and cardamom for warming and soothing.

o Lemon verbena and lemon balm to refresh and relax.

Flower essences

o **Female Essence** – a ready-made blend of flower essences to support the female system.

o **Flower remedies** (such as Bach): especially: **Impatiens** (for impatient feelings) **Holly** (for when you're feeling prickly) and **Oak** (for strength).

Essential Oils

Can be used for burning, massage or in a bath – should always be used diluted in a base oil (e.g. sweet almond oil) if applied direct to the skin:

o **Clary Sage** – brings clarity to the mind.

o **Rose** – good for anger.

o **Geranium** – good for depression and stress.

o **Neroli** – good for soothing, weepiness and depression.

o **Mandarin/Orange** – uplifting.

o **Juniper** – diuretic for bloating and swelling.

o **Lavender** – calming, good for migraines.

o **Chamomile** – calming.

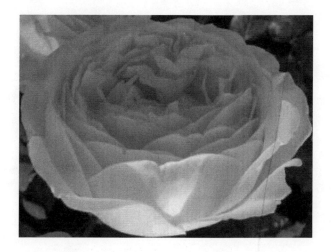

Cream

o **Natural Progesterone** – made from **wild yam** good for PMT, menopause, cramps and migraine. Applied to the breasts or abdomen daily.

Nutritional healing

Eat well, dear woman – do not starve yourself. Your body needs to be fed. It is good and right to eat well. Find which foods work for **your** body. Find your own rhythms for eating – and be aware that these might not be what those around you need, nor what you were brought up with.

Honour your body with every mouthful you take. Find your own levels of enough. Discover your own levels of satisfaction. Be aware of destructive eating patterns which you may have developed – eating instead of expressing, or even feeling, your emotions, or dosing yourself with caffeine rather than resting.

o   Keep hydrated – drink lots of water and herbal tea.

o   Water or fresh apple juice with fresh lemon juice, grated garlic and ginger is a powerful tonic to support and cleanse the liver.

o   Many women swear by green smoothies to boost energy, especially during moon time. Add a large handful of leafy greens (spinach, kale, lettuce and perhaps some spirulina) to your normal smoothie base of banana and juice, blend and serve.

o   Consider taking supplements of B vitamins, especially B6 and B12, iron, zinc and magnesium, especially leading up to menstruation, if you are breastfeeding or if you are vegetarian.

o   Zinc relieves cramps. It can be found in dark green vegetables, wild plants, seaweeds and nuts.

o   Eat lots of green leafy vegetables and dried fruits for iron to ensure you are not anaemic.

o   High protein foods such as meat, dairy, seeds, fish and chocolate contain tryptophan – a mood boosting amino acid.

o   The caffeine and sugar in chocolate lift your spirits – but they can also be migraine inducing, so watch out!

o   Cut back on (or eliminate!) alcohol, sugar, caffeine and processed foods if you find this improves PMT symptoms.

o   Many women find that they have added cravings for simple carbohydrates and meat approaching their moon time.

o   Some suggest that eating red meat at this time can make your bleeding heavier.

In everything you eat – honour yourself.

In every rest you take – honour yourself.

In how you spend your time – honour yourself.

In the people you spend your time with – honour yourself.

In nourishing your body and soul with love and mindful awareness, you learn to truly honour everyone and everything that your life touches.

9

THE SEASONS OF WOMANHOOD

In our culture we have no formal way of celebrating the seasons of our lives as women. Part of my work is in re-instigating and re-imagining the sacred celebrations of womanhood. These important steps on our paths and in our cycles go unmarked, and so we may believe that they do not matter. But they do. And it is up to us to find a way to fully acknowledge and celebrate them. This might be in an informal ceremony alone or a more elaborate celebration with a group of women friends.

A ceremony is a formal way of welcoming a new phase and mourning or releasing an old phase. It is a making sacred of our bodies and their functions, and making meaning of our personal journey. If we do not do this we can often get ill or depressed, as our minds remain stuck in the past or skipping forwards into the future whilst our bodies are here in the present doing their body-thing!

In this book we look in depth at celebrating menarche and our monthly bleed. A future book will go into depth in how to celebrate pregnancy and motherhood.

Female rites to celebrate:

o   menarche (first period)

o   loss of virginity

o   monthly cycle

o   birthday

o   marriage or pair-bonding

o   pregnancy

o   miscarriage

o   abortion

o   impending birth (mother blessing)

o   birth

o   establishment of breastfeeding

o   re-commencement of menstruation after birth

o   conscious end of childbearing

o   weaning

o   commencement of menopause

o   last bleed

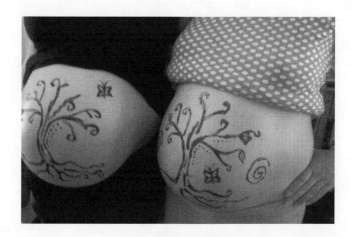

And you...

Which of these have you or do you celebrate already?

Do you feel the lack of not having celebrated any of these in the past?

Which would you like to celebrate in the future?

Are there any of your friends or family who are at an important stage in their lives that you would like to help them to celebrate?

How might you do this?

10

MENARCHE
THE FIRST BLOOD

The reactions of the people close to a girl as she approaches her first period, is carried in her psyche. Whether we celebrate or denigrate her determines the next several years of her life - her adolescent identity. These same circumstances subtly influence all succeeding physical emotional and psychological passages for the rest of her life.

If she is joyously celebrated, she moves into adolescence self-confident and proud of herself as a budding woman. If she is made to feel ashamed of her body, she feels tainted with the shame and self-loathing for being female.

Virginia Beane Rutter, *Celebrating Girls*

In the process of becoming ourselves more fully, it is crucial to reclaim our own stories and experiences, for in them we will find the seeds of healing.

Now that we have our own language for our bodies, and an understanding of our cycles, let us go deeper in our work, to excavate our lives and find what lies beneath the surface. Let us enter our own stories and reclaim our truth and power from them. After bringing our stories into our present, the next chapter will offer the framework, and a living example of how to celebrate your entry into womanhood anew – full of love, acceptance and celebration.

My story

The first time I found out about periods was at school. Just before leaving junior school each girl child was issued with a little pocket-sized booklet entitled *Personally Yours*. I still remember the cover, a fuzzy anonymous image of a reclining girl with a blonde bob, pink jumper and jeans. We were intrigued. We took them outside at lunch break and three of us girlfriends lay on our backs, legs up to the ceiling in a concrete crawling tunnel in the playing field, and devoured this new information. We were fascinated, not disgusted in any way. I remember thinking many years later that it was cunning marketing. The booklets were compiled by Tampax. Of course they reassured us that we could still swim or ride a horse: just use a tampon. I was reassured. It felt exciting, but calm.

For me it was to be three years before I experienced it for myself. I remember being in my flute lesson. I felt muddle-headed, clumsy, frustrated, and very vulnerable. I cried and cried. My poor, male teacher, was as kind and understanding as he could be, I was obviously just having a "bad day". I went to the toilet after the lesson. And there, to my astonishment was copious red blood on the toilet paper. I felt excited– a sense of knowing that this was a big deal for me, for my life. A shift, a change had happened. School was over for the day. But it was a boarding school so I would not be seeing any of my family until the weekend. It felt momentous. I needed to share that I was changed. I grabbed my best friend, and again we went outside. We walked in the gardens and I told her. It felt so right to share it with a female friend, and to do it out in nature.

But being in boarding school also had its downsides. I felt a deep shame. I didn't want anyone else to know that I had my period. So I set up elaborate

94

coughing routines when I opened the crinkly sanitary towel wrapper. I spent ages scouring knickers from leaks, and eventually settled on black underwear all the time.

Only trusted friends knew when you were "on". We used to watch each other's backs, literally. In the summer term we wore white and blue striped skirts which showed leaks very easily. It was a sisterhood. We had a special code word: "P", which then, for reasons unknown to me, became "Mr P". Then because my father was Mr P, we called our periods "Stephen", after my dad. What irony to have a male period, though we didn't see that at the time!

My mother cried when I told her. And I told my step mother too. They were both lovely and so good with any practical questions I had, there was no awkwardness. I swore my step mother to secrecy – she was, after all, the sisterhood. But at some point, my father figured out that I was menstruating, and was hurt that I had not told him. I got a five page letter from him expressing this. What business is my blood of yours? I wondered. I felt vulnerable for having my privacy, my secrecy, broken, and by a man.

And so it continues to this day. My trusted sisterhood knows about my cycles – it gives them insight into "where I'm at", but I find it more difficult to tell my husband and children. It feels like a sacred secret, which I don't trust them so much with. For my sisters, they know, they understand, they truly get it, because they've got it too!

And you...

Have you told the story of your first time – perhaps you would like to do it in your journal, at a menarche celebration for yourself, on your blog, to your daughter, to a close friend, at a women's group, in a red tent – honour your experience.

What did you wish could have been different? Can you make that right for yourself now?

OOO

Medicated moon time

My moon time in my teens was hard. Not only did I have the mood swings of teenage girlhood and PMT, but my period pains were so bad that I would often faint in the first couple of days of menstruation. I would be writhing in agony, often on bed rest with a hot water bottle and as many pain killers as I could safely take.

I was a high achiever, with full busy days at school. The mentality around periods was that they got you off swimming, but that was it – carry on regardless, they shouldn't have any impact on you. And so I tried to do that for years.

The doctor prescribed me Ponstan at first, which had little effect. He then placed me on the contraceptive pill. I was 16 and proud to be "on the Pill". Looking back now that makes me feel angry that there was no other way of helping me to deal with this.

I felt sad, depressed, as though I was floating below the surface of life. I didn't feel like myself on the Pill but no one would take me seriously, no one told me it was because I was cut off from my own rhythm.

Looking back I mourn those lost years of unmedicated girlhood, of my sexuality blossoming unhindered by chemical interference. I am angry about the potential lifelong side effects which went unmentioned. I am sad that I trusted the doctors.

And you...

Have you ever been on the Pill?

How was it for you?

Did you have side effects?

What were they?

Why did you go onto it? And what made you come off it?

How might you share your knowledge with other girls and women?

Book review

The Pill: Are you sure it's for you?

Jane Bennett & Alexandra Pope

Having seen this book reviewed when it was first published, a couple of years back, I took note, but never bought it because, being in the midst of baby making, I was no longer on the Pill, nor, intending to be again. I had had a miserable experience on it, trading its contraceptive function for my own libido, increased migraines, weight gain and generally feeling "not me". I refused to go on it again.

It was in starting The Happy Womb that I decided that I needed to read this book to see if it would be of use to my readers.

My advice? Get yourself a copy this instant.

*The scientific research on the impacts of the Pill in this book is revelatory. The authors examine every angle: physical, emotional, short term and long term that the Pill has on women and their cycles. It shares the experiences of hundreds women from around the world and makes you see that not only are **you not alone** if you experience a lot of the "minimal side effects" of the Pill, but actually **you are in the majority.** In fact, fully one third of Pill users stop taking it because of depression. It added hard evidence to my own personal experience of the Pill which doctors ignored, denied or belittled.*

*Some of the effects are scary, especially those which are permanent in your body. Your levels of globulin, which binds testosterone and affects libido, are four times lower, **forever**, if you have taken the Pill. You have a doubled risk of breast and ovarian cancer if you took it under the age of twenty. Ditto brittle bones. All things I wished someone had told me then.*

It is clearly written, full of easily digestible facts and research. The first half focuses on issues with the Pill – from depression to weight gain, loss of libido, infertility, thrombosis – the second half focuses on other forms of contraception and ways to attune to your cycle. It is a gold mine of both scientific knowledge and women's wisdom.

This would be top of my list of books to give to all young women.

OOO

Celebrating menarche

If you feel that your entry into womanhood was lacking and that this still has an impact on your attitude towards your moon time or your female body, it is never too late: create a menarche celebration for yourself now!

If you are a mother of daughters you may want to allow the idea of how to celebrate their entry to womanhood to gently percolate for a few years so that when the time comes you are not caught off-guard, unsure of how to respond.

If you create your own menarche celebration then you will not only be serving yourself in healing and acceptance, but also the women whom you involve in the planning and celebration. Furthermore it will allow you to develop your vision for how you might celebrate your daughter when her time comes.

By creating your own celebration first there will be no sense of jealousy of your daughter for having what you never had. Instead when her time comes, it will be a pure offering of love for her and an embracing of her, rather than offering her something that you wish for yourself, which, if it is rejected or scorned, will feel doubly hurtful. And in this awareness of her as the virgin and you the mother, you will be able to both stand in your own power, in your own places in the circle.

It is important to remember the sense of vulnerability we feel at puberty about our bodies, and the need for privacy. Do not impose a celebration on your daughter, rather celebrate her as she is, in a way which makes her feel special and loved, not in the way that you would have wanted, or an intricate ceremony that the books suggest. Allow for the fact that although you might want to share your wisdom, she might not want to hear it!

Before embarking on planning a menarche celebration, take some time to reflect – either in thought or by journaling your responses to the following queries:

o   Why do you want to celebrate her menarche?

o   How do you want her to feel?

o How does she feel about her period?

o How is your relationship with her at the moment?

o How would you like it to be?

o How was your relationship with your mother at her age?

o How is it now?

o Does she have a godmother whom she is close to? If not this might be a good time to (between you) appoint one to her to help her navigate these potentially turbulent few years.

o Are you at peace with your own menarche? If not, what do you need for yourself firstly?

o Has she ever experienced – either first-hand, or through hearing you talk – any sacred feminine ceremonies? If she, or you both, are beginners to this, be very mindful of your comfort zones.

Before planning anything, be sure to **clarify your intention** – everything you plan should have the express and implicit intention of making her feel:

o appreciated

o included

o loved

o accepted

o special

o grown up

o welcomed into your circle of women

We often try to keep our precious babies as little girls. Use her menarche celebration to show that she is growing into a woman and that you honour and respect that.

If she has a godmother or aunt who is close, why not involve her in the planning? If she doesn't this might be a good opportunity to appoint a godmother/ moon mother/ mentor. This woman (perhaps a friend of yours, or a mother of one of her friends) is asked to act as her official friend and mentor through her teen years when she may not feel able to approach you, but needs the advice of an older woman whom she (and you) respects and trusts. We all need many mothers in our lifetimes – let her know that this is OK with you.

This is also a good time to tell her about fertility, her cycles and perhaps more about sex. To connect what objective knowledge she has to her own body, to share with her the reality of her own potential to nurture life, and with it the responsibilities. This must of course be guided very much by her own level of maturity and your family's beliefs: a girl reaching her menarche at nine is at a very different place in her personal and sexual development to one who is fourteen.

You might also choose to celebrate with an intimate circle of friends and family. Or to share the celebration with other girls of the same age. Perhaps you would both feel more at ease with a one-to-one celebration. You might choose to involve others in this by asking your close friends and family to send her gifts, letters and special quotations which you can present her with in private when her day of bleeding comes. Judge it according to her feelings of sociability and comfort in groups or with intimacy.

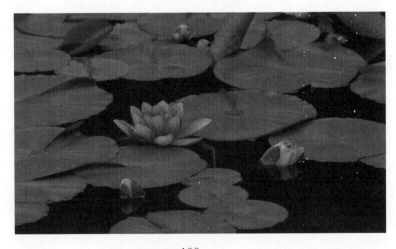

Activities to celebrate your daughter's menarche
This is a list of possible activities – you do not need to try to do them all!

o write her a letter

o get her ears pierced

o or a daring new haircut

o give her a moon journal

o take her out to dinner

o have a special dinner at home

o give her flowers

o make a cake

o buy her her own red towels

o make or buy her her own pouch for sanitary towels

o give her her first handbag

o or a beautiful piece of jewellery to mark the occasion

o make her up with lipstick, Kohl and bright nail polish

All of these activities seek to welcome her into the world of women, doing and sharing "grown up" activities with her as a means of loving acceptance into the next stage of her life's journey.

As her mother you might want to share with her your memories of:

o your first period,

o being a teenager,

o your pregnancy with her and her birth (or adoption).

You might also want to vocalise:

- o your hopes and wishes for her in her life,

- o an acknowledgement of her growing beauty, power and spirit,

- o a conscious letting go of her as your little girl and an embracing of her as a young woman forging her own life.

All of this is a part of passing on narratives to the next generation, passing forward their own stories, which we have acted as story-keepers for until this point. And of course, it is another breaking of the female silence.

Also crucially important at this time is for mothers of boys to find a way to gently and lovingly educate their sons into the mysteries of a woman's body and her cycles, to give him an accurate and respectful understanding of female fertility which he will take out into the world with him.

It is vital that we talk with other mothers about preparing our sons and daughters for adulthood. It is not just "your problem". We are all in the same boat, and all hold part of the answer. So pool your resources, work within your own community to find ways to give meaning, and meaningful information, to your children who are coming of age.

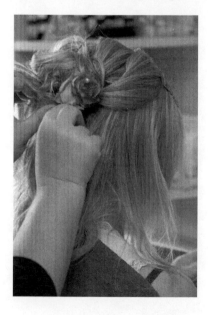

Menarche celebration

Simple steps for creating your own sacred menarche celebration...

o Invite a circle of women to celebrate with you – your mother, sisters, friends, daughters...

o Decorate the space beautifully – red and white flowers, candles, inspiring pictures, drapes, incense – make it feel special and sacred.

o Dress in red or white to celebrate bleeding and fertility.

o Have a special welcome – perhaps walking under branches, or over scattered rose petals. Have your hands and feet washed with rose water and your hair brushed.

o Sit in a circle according to where you are now in your cycle.

o Have a reading of an empowering women's myth (see *Red Moon, Thirteen Moons, Women who Run with the Wolves* for resources).

o Tell stories of your first bleeding, how it felt, what it meant, how it was received.

o Have your head adorned with red ochre, or your hands or belly painted in henna.

o Join hands and sing or chant.

o Each create a red necklace or bracelet which you can wear to remember this day.

o Light a candle of blessing for yourself.

o Share food afterwards to ground the energy – you might choose red foods and fruits to symbolise fertility.

OOO

Menarche: A journey into womanhood

by Rachael Hertogs

Rites of passage have begun to reappear in our society as we recognise the importance of honouring our young people and guiding them gently into adulthood. Ceremonies, vision quests, men's and women's lodges, rite of passage courses, festivals and camps are becoming more and more popular.

I have been working with women and their daughters for many years supporting them in celebrating their rite of passage.

The first period is known as menarche. Tribal traditions have celebrated menarche for thousands of years. Some rituals include the whole tribe, others are more private, shared amongst close women friends and family. Some are quite extreme, including genital mutilation, cutting, scarring and tattooing, whilst others are more gentle – being fed, massaged and sung to.

I believe how a young woman is guided through this experience can affect her for the rest of her life.

A modern menarche celebration

I have been taking part in the menarche ceremony preparation at Sacred Arts Camp for a number of years – running workshops with the young women and their mothers; teaching them about charting their cycle; making moon necklaces; decorating red and white candles...

What I love about this ceremony is that it is open to any woman who hadn't been celebrated at her menarche, as well as all the girls who have recently begun to bleed. So ages of those taking part can be from ten to forty! It also involves the men, the grandmothers, the very young girls – anyone who wants to join in can have a role.

All week women meet in my moon lodge tipi to co-create the ceremony – deciding what songs will be sung, what dances to dance, finding musicians, collecting red and white clothes for the women taking part, choosing who will take which role....

Meanwhile the young women choose a Moon Mother who will attend the ceremony with them holding their hand and reassuring them, bringing them a gift, helping them to get ready, they might share blood stories with them and as part of the ceremony they dream them a 'moon name' the night before the ritual.

Many Moon Mother/Moon Daughter relationships continue years after the ceremony – even though girls may choose a woman who they only see once a year at camp! They also choose a Moon Father – someone older who can be another 'wise father figure' in their life and who will also make them a crown of leaves and flowers for the ceremony! The Moon Fathers have a powerful role in the ritual: bringing in the male energy.

Other men of the community get involved too. They meet to prepare – perhaps creating a song for the ceremony, as well as sharing stories with each other about men's traditions and honouring women. Their part in the ceremony is to 'guard' the sacred ceremonial space by dressing as 'warriors' and walking around the outside perimeter whilst drumming and chanting.

The ceremony

Each year the ceremony is slightly different. The ritual begins with the decorating of the space. Our big top is draped with whatever cloths and sheets we have, flowers are placed in vases and jars, an entrance is made from willow and flowers. We light candles and incense and raise the energy by singing and chanting while we decorate and smudge ourselves with white sage!

All the women dress up: white if they haven't begun to bleed yet, red if they're a bleeding woman and black/purple for the menopausal women.

While this is happening the young women get ready with their Moon Mothers in the moon lodge, being anointed with sacred water and dressing in white, with a white ribbon in their hair.

Walking in to a big top filled with over two hundred women singing is a powerful experience! They sang and danced for the girls and their Moon

Mothers, and then we left to change the girls from white to red. As each one left the space, they turned and called out their name symbolizing leaving their 'girl-child' part of themselves behind.

While we helped them change in the moon lodge, the ceremony continued with the passing of the 'yoni cushion' as a talking stick. As it was passed, each woman who held it spoke three words to summarise their bleeding experience, words like: connected, pain, loss, renewal and even "I'm not pregnant!"

After that songs and chants are shared until the young women re-enter, dressed in beautiful red clothes. The singing continues in honour of them and then there is the ceremonial hair cutting – once again symbolising the letting go of their childhood. The hair with the white ribbon is cut away and they are anointed with a red ochre crescent moon on their forehead, to remind them of their moon connection and the rhythm and flow of the moon. They drank from the sacred goblet (blackcurrant juice!) and then the Moon Mothers step forward to bless them with gifts and their new 'moon names' are whispered to them.

Now is the time for the men to enter! The Grandmothers have been guarding the entrance the whole time and now step back to allow the men in. But first they are challenged: 'Do you come in to this space with love and respect for your sisters?' To which of course they answered yes!

The 'Moon Fathers' stepped forward and crowned their Moon Daughters, as the rest of the men sang their gift song they had composed. In return, our gift to the men for protecting our space was to share with them a blood mystery story, told by one of our amazing storytellers. After that the musicians played, joined by the drummers and it was time to celebrate and dance the evening away!

The young women left with their Moon Mums to go back to the moon lodge and have chocolate cake and to ground themselves after the ritual. Later that night (it was a full moon) we had a women's sweat lodge – the perfect ending to a wonderful day!

(Reprinted with the author's permission. A longer version of this article first appeared in **JUNO** magazine in 2010.)

Rachael runs a UK based website, Moontimes, which sells cloth menstrual pads, books and a whole host of products related to menstruation. She has produced a booklet entitled Menarche- a Journey into Womanhood which includes articles and stories about menarche, ideas for celebrations, tips for connecting to and charting your cycle, book recommendations, poems and much more. She is also the creatress of the yoni cushion mentioned in the ritual- see her website for photos!

www.moontimes.co.uk

www.rachaelhertogs.co.uk

www.sacredartscamp.org

11

HONOURING OUR MOON TIME

Any cycling woman knows the deep yearning for quietude during her flow time. Every ounce of our body and soul calls for rest, while our culture calls us to keep going, no matter what.

DeAnna L'am, menstrual educator

In *The Pill: Are you sure it's for you?* the authors refer to "menstruation as meditation" pointing out that it is our own personal Sabbath. In Miranda Gray's *Red Moon* she observes that we live by solar months consisting of man-made "working weeks" divided by regular periods of rest, "weekends". Whereas a woman's natural pattern is three weeks on and one week off. If you added together the weekend-days in a lunar month you would have the five days needed to rest and reset, rebalance and regroup during your moon time! It is, as they say, still a man's world.

Our culture does not honour the Sabbath, a real day of rest, as our ancestors did. Nor do we have dispensation to "take it easy" during our moon time from the outside world, as the Native Americans and ancient Canaanite women did.

Often when we rest all sorts of uncomfortable feelings can come up (and comments get made). We might feel:

o   lazy

o   like we ought to be doing something

o   that we're wasting time

o   guilty

o   bored

In my own experience creating space for moon time rest and retreat is vital for my mental health. If I do not and try to carry on as normal I get exhausted, physically and mentally, I get resentful and angry. If I am on my feet for most of the day, or doing exercise on the first two days of my cycle I get crampy too, and my flow seems even heavier. I feel literally dragged down. Many would recognise these symptoms as PMT. But I have found that if I honour my moon time these symptoms alleviate, if not totally disappear.

Your moon time is the time when you are feeling tiredest, slowest, when your energy is reflective, when your body needs rest, and your mind needs quiet. Creating a retreat space for yourself allows you to honour your body's natural energy cycle.

We all need to create time and space for:

o   retreat

o   self-care

o   rest

o   reflection

Both SARK and Leonie Dawson from Goddess Guidebooks talk about writing ourselves permission slips for what we really need and want. Just like the permission slip that your mother might have written to get you off swimming when you had your period.

…...

Dearest …..................................... (fill in your name)

I give you my total permission to
…..............................(whatever it is you give permission for)
for the whole of today/ this week/ this month/ forever!

With all my love

…..................................... (fill in your name)

....

May I gently suggest that you get into the habit of giving yourself permission
– and actively write one for yourself.

If this is too challenging for you, then take it one baby step at a time. Just like
learning to speak a new language, or to play an instrument, keep doing a little
bit. So perhaps today allow yourself to sit and dream for five minutes. Or to
go to bed half an hour earlier than usual. Or to write in your journal for five
minutes. Just choose one of those things. Then tomorrow, or next month,
you can build up to two of them, and so on, until learning to make time for
rest comes more naturally to you.

And you…

How do you create mindfulness in your day? Perhaps yoga, tai chi,
meditation, a walk, prayer, some journaling time...

How might you simplify your life during your moon time?

What little acts feel comforting to you?

Retreat

In the next chapter I will be sharing how to create a sacred space to share with other women to celebrate your moon time. But before we co-create with (and for) others, we need this practice to be rooted for and in ourselves. The rest of this chapter will take you through how to create a safe, sanctuary space, a private moon lodge just for you.

Often when we think of retreats, we think of disappearing to a beautiful hut high in the hills, or to a religious order, or an expensive spa. But learning how to retreat within the confines of our own lives is a vital lesson for us to learn as women.

The most important part of retreat is creating a space apart from everyone, where you will be uninterrupted. Many women refer to it as "retreating to their cave" – think seclusion, dark, quiet, containment and safety.

In practical terms this means picking both the right time of day, and a place that you can shut a door to. I usually use our bedroom, both when the younger children are sleeping during the day, and then again in the evening as soon as they have gone to bed. (I must point out at this juncture that I have had a baby co-sleeping in my bed for the past six years, so if I retreat in the evening time, it is done with baby in there!)

Or perhaps you can tempt your partner to head out with friends to the bar or cinema so you can use your main living area below.

Whichever space you use, be sure to make it feel safe. Ensure that you will not be burst in upon or have demands made upon you or judgements made.

Do what you can,

with what you have,

where you are!

Shut the door, draw the curtains, take the phone off the hook, turn off your computer and commit to not answering the door.

111

Make your space feel **womb-like, safe and contained**.

Cover up anything which is messy or distracting with a sheet or beautiful throw: the TV, kids' toys, paperwork, general mess…

I suggest **gentle lighting**, like that which you might see in any sacred space such as a church or birthing room. Either a single lamp, or candles. This lowering of light levels has a direct impact on brain function and hormone levels. This helps you to shift into a more relaxed, peaceful and intuitive frame of mind and helps you to feel like you have had a real rest.

Perhaps you might like to **burn incense or essential oils**, or massage your hands and feet with a sweet smelling cream. **Scent is a powerful way to set a sacred space.**

Your set up can be as simple or ceremonially intricate as your heart desires.

Make a **hot water bottle**, hot pad, castor oil pack or just wrap yourself in a snuggly blanket to keep you cosy and soothe your aches.

Get yourself a big glass of water or herbal tea. Hold it in your hands and drink mindfully from it. This will help to get you back into your body, and to replace the fluids that you are losing through your menstruation.

Consciously breathe to centre yourself. Allow yourself to settle back into your body and the whirl of the day to slow to a stop. Allow the two spheres – your inner and outer selves – to come into alignment, otherwise you will be coming from a place of mental chatter, or emotional turmoil. Sit for as long as it takes to allow this to settle.

If it helps you, **do a guided meditation** (perhaps the happy womb visualisation on www.thehappywomb.com).

For mothers or busy working women, these acts alone, especially the conscious delineation of your own physical space, which you so rarely have, is a powerful tool in taking back your own energy and power. It teaches you, and those you share your life with, about your desire to set limits on others' demands on you during your moon time. Setting out your space is a conscious way of signalling that you need to be alone and that it is sacred and to be respected.

However if you want more to "do" then I have a wonderful smorgasbord of activities to suggest to you – but, as always, don't try to do them all!

Activities

Journaling

Try journaling whatever comes up in your head: don't plan, rationalise or be too clever. Perhaps write in free verse. I find quite often that the "voice" which emerges during my moon time is a poetic voice rather than rational linear thought. It speaks directly to me and I sit and transcribed its rich images.

Moon letters

A dear friend and I wrote moon letters over the course of a year. Every moon time we would sit and write a handwritten letter – we shared our dreams, visions for the month ahead, reflections, quotes from books, poems we had written. These were our way into reconnecting with our own cycles, sharing our wisdom and insight, learning to take time out from the demands of being mothers to young children. It deepened our friendship at a time when we both struggled to find the time, space and energy to talk on the phone.

Dream journaling

Our moon time is often a time of powerful archetypal dreams which can stay with us through the day. By keeping a journal we tap into this wisdom, we find messages from a deeper level of consciousness, and begin to be able to interpret the symbols and themes of our own personal dream language. In learning to honour our dreams, we also honour our need to sleep!

Self-care regime

Now is a great time to enjoy nourishing self-care practices – perhaps a face mask or manicure. Take time to brush your hair or moisturise your skin – nurture and care for your physical body.

Meditation/ trance/ prayer

Meditation needn't be a formal practice. Simply slowing the mind, whilst watching a candle flame, or spiralling steam coming from a cup of tea, gazing at the moon out of the window, or listening to the wind whistling – all of these bring us into a receptive meditative state where we just are, and our mind can let go of control. Meditation is seen as listening to the divine whereas prayer is active, talking to the divine. The divine might be your god or goddess, the universe or your highest sense of self.

Creative doodling/ imaginative painting/ collage

Any creative activities that can be done in a dreamlike state, which do not require deep concentration or planning, but are rather an exploration of colour, materials and mood, are what is called for at moon time.

Focus on creative work which is expressive and non-productive – this is especially important if you are a working artist – this is not a time to finish your latest commission, but rather a time to mine your unconscious for images.

I have recently discovered SoulCollage by Seena B. Frost, which is a wonderful visual technique for creating your own archetype/ tarot type cards which would be a great moon time project.

Tarot/ angel cards/ runes/ dowsing

Tap into your heightened intuitive powers at this time with whatever intuitive practice you feel comfortable with.

Reading

Now is the time to immerse yourself in a book which feeds your soul – perhaps something spiritual or meaningful to you as a woman. In your menstrual phase you are especially sensitive, so stay away from horror or thrillers which can overload you emotionally.

Whatever you choose to do, take this opportunity to fill yourself full to the brim with love, inspiration, gentleness and beauty.

Daily self-care rituals for moon time

If you do not feel called to create a retreat for yourself, the bare minimum you should do at your moon time is some extra special self-care – this might include:

o   Special underwear.

o   Dark pyjamas and clothes.

o   Snuggly socks or jumper.

o   Red towels.

o   A manicure/ pedicure/ facial/ massage/ hot stone treatment.

o   A moon time necklace or shawl or ring to signal to those who know that you are bleeding.

o   Showers rather than bath (see below).

o   Menstrual products that really work for you – perhaps beautiful cloth ones, a moon cup or thick night pads.

o   A cup of tea (see below).

OOO

Healing with water

Water is the representative element for women – fluid, ever-changing, sometimes calm and reflective, sometimes turbulent and dangerous. If you are feeling unsettled water is often the most balancing element to restore you to yourself. Just as the moon most strongly influences our flows, so it influences all water on the planet – the tides and even the water uptake of plants.

Water can be used therapeutically in many different ways:

o   we can take it in through our senses – a walk on the beach or by a river

o   sitting by a waterfall or garden water feature

o   immersion by swimming, showering or sacred bathing

o   imbibing it – through drinking tea, soup or just a big glass of water

o   steam – through inhalation, in a sauna or simply for contemplation

Below I share with you two ways of transforming the simple acts of tea drinking and bathing into sacred and mindful practices, which bring calm and relaxation to your day and give you a little breathing space, even in the busiest of lives.

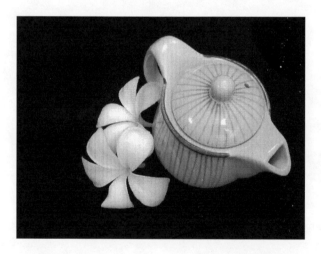

Tea ceremony

As a busy woman, ordinary days can often spiral out of control making you feel exhausted and frazzled. Around your moon time this can be totally overwhelming.

Many people drink tea as a refreshment, and for many their tea times are a way of getting through the day – the combination of caffeine, liquid and a much needed break revives them. My mother is one of life's tea drinkers; I however am not. I came to tea drinking late in life and still I don't enjoy a traditional cuppa with milk and sugar. It was my time in Japan that brought home to me the ceremonial aspects of tea drinking, whilst the wise woman tradition established the healing reasons for taking time to drink herbal tea.

So if you have a full day and really can't off load any tasks, then the tea ceremony is a centring, healing way of taking time out within a normal day, helping to recharge you mentally and physically.

How to do it
o   Firstly, give yourself permission to take 10-15 minutes for yourself. The tea ceremony can be done with others, but the temptation is to chat and the calming, soothing energy is dissipated.

o   If you can expose yourself to a natural element whilst doing the tea ceremony, the healing, calming effect will be magnified. If it is a fine day then sit outside. Or if you have a conservatory or some indoor plants in your office, sit there and absorb the earth energy. If it is a blustery day like today as I'm writing this, sit by an open fire and absorb the fire energy.

o   Turn off your phone and do your best to ensure that you will not be interrupted.

o   From the moment you turn on the tap to fill the kettle, or enter the cafe, imagine you are drawing a comforting bubble around yourself. Nothing, bar an emergency will enter this and disturb you.

o   Still your mind as the kettle boils. Close your eyes and take a few deep, aware breaths. Choose your cup and tea according to your intuition – what do you need right now? Perhaps a pretty cup to lift your feminine spirits, or a hand-made earthenware mug which feels solid and comforting. What tea do you need? (See the chapter on Herbal Healing for a selection of nourishing women's teas.)

o   Pour the water over the herbs or tea bag and as you leave it to steep, watch the steam spiralling upwards. Allow your thoughts and spirit to soar upwards with it, light, free and unbounded. Breathe consciously and deeply and allow your body to settle and rest. Check in with each part of your body from your toes to your head and relax any tension.

o   When your tea is ready, cradle the cup in your hands, feel the warmth. Inhale the aroma of the tea deeply. And mindfully take your first sip. Allow yourself to savour the taste, to really experience all the sensations of flavour, warmth, moisture, as they enter your body and infuse you. With each mindful sip allow your tiredness to seep away and a sense of calm energy fill you.

o   Take a few moments before you are finished to bring to mind something you are grateful for. I always finish my tea ceremony by being grateful for the water which makes my tea, the herbs which grew in the earth, the healing herbal knowledge of people and the time to reconnect with myself.

o   Take your mindfulness, your calm, your soothed body gently back into your day.

Sacred bathing

Cultures around the world have used sacred bathing as a means of purification after menstruation – from Orthodox Jews to the Japanese. Using candles, heady essential oils or cascades of bubbles, relaxing music and a big fluffy towel transform a normal hygiene routine into a ritual fit for Cleopatra. I was reawakened to sacred bathing recently by Shonagh Home's *Ix Chel Mysteries: 7 Teachings from the Mayan Sacred Feminine*.

I don't like to take baths during my moon time. I have showers and then a sacred, purifying bath when my bleeding has finished. This is another form of steam meditation and water therapy, and one which I look forward to every month.

How to do it

o   Firstly, give yourself permission to take 30 minutes for yourself.

o Turn off your phone. If you have children, make sure they are being cared for so that you do not need to be distracted. Occasionally I have managed to do this with children in tow – in which case set them up with an activity – perhaps filling cups in the sink where you can see them. Close the door so you know they are in with you and safe.

o From the moment you turn on the tap imagine you are drawing a comforting bubble around yourself. Nothing, bar an emergency will enter this and disturb you.

o Still your mind as the bath runs. Close your eyes and take a few deep, aware breaths. What scents do you need? Do you want bubbles or oils (be aware that the two do not work together!) Perhaps strew some flower petals on the water.

- Clary sage – brings clarity to the mind

- Lavender – calming

- Rose – good for anger

- Geranium – calming

- Neroli – soothing, good for weepiness and depression

- Mandarin/ orange – uplifting

- Juniper – diuretic for bloating and swelling

- Chamomile – calming

o Make it as hot as you can and as deep as you can. This is a bath for luxuriating in. Be grateful that you have the water and fuel to be able to do this, hold in mind other women in the world who do not and perhaps send some love and blessings their way.

o Light some candles and dim or turn off the lights.

- Choose some relaxing music, an empowering teacher's CD, an audio guided meditation. Or maybe just silence.

- Leave your fluffy towel, bath robe, clean clothes or pyjamas warming on a nearby heater. And have some slippers there too!

- As you take off your clothes imagine you are taking off the suffering of the day. Look with love at your body.

- Ease yourself gently into the bath. Lie back, take a deep breath and close your eyes! Imagine that you are contained within a loving, nurturing womb.

- After a while, open your eyes and adjust to the dim light. Allow yourself to really experience all the sensations of scent, warmth, moisture, as they surround your body and infuse you.

- Watch the steam spiralling upwards. Allow your thoughts and spirit to soar upwards with it, light, free and unbounded. Breathe consciously and deeply and allow your body to settle and rest. Check in with each part of your body from your toes to your head and consciously relax any tension.

- Gently and lovingly wash yourself from top to toe with a special loofah or sponge and some indulgent shower gel or exfoliant. Be appreciative of each and every part of your body as you wash it.

- Take your time emerging from the bath so as not to be light headed. Dry yourself with loving care and attention. Moisturise or oil your skin and brush your hair.

- Take your mindfulness, your calm, your soothed body gently back into your day, being sure not to catch cold.

12

RED TENTS & MOON LODGES

At best, the Red Tent Temple times are like homecomings for us.

ALisa Starkweather, foundress of the Red Tent Temple Movement

A place where women are allowed to Be rather than continually Do...

DeAnna L'am, menstrual educator

Around the world a new consciousness is springing up, a yearning to honour our female experience and to create new rituals to replace those long ago lost.

The red tent is one such idea that seems to resonate strongly with many women. In sharing the concept of red tents and moon lodges, I hope to inspire you to create your own. With that in mind, I want to share with you variety of voices from around the world, brave souls who are visioning a more beautiful, creative, empowered way of being a woman.

What is a red tent?

The idea of the **red tent** was introduced by Anita Diamant in her book *The Red Tent*, published in 1997. She brings to life a group of central women figures in the Bible whose lives were glossed over by male Old Testament authors. She re-imagines the old Canaanite ways in the time of Abraham, where women who were menstruating or about to give birth were secluded for a few days in a red tent. There they would bleed onto the earth and be relieved of all domestic responsibilities. This was where they shared their wisdom, cared for themselves and each other and initiated girls into the rites of womanhood.

A **moon lodge** or **bleeding lodge** is a similar idea, but comes from the Native American tradition. It is a place that a woman goes to descend into her depths during her moon time, to be still and experience the magic available to her at this time.

"When women started to bleed, they left their homes and families to go to the sacred introspective space of the Bleeding Lodge. The Lodge was honoured and respected by the entire community, for the dreams and visions of the bleeding women brought vital survival information such as planting and healing knowledge and guidance on community relations. When there were questions that needed to be answered, the women would go to the Lodge and ask the Ancestors. All questions were always answered by the Ancient Ancestors. The entire community benefited through the powerful gifts of the women's bleeding cycle.

Since our Ancient Grandmothers probably all bled together, many women shared the Womb Lodge at one time. Ceremonies to honour our womb cycles, celebrate the cycles of the Earth and Moon, and rites of passage were developed by these women from visions and dreams during their bleeding times in the Sacred Lodge. These traditions were passed down in the initiatory rites of the Blood Lodge from mother to daughter."

Songs of Bleeding by *Spider*

"Since ancient times women have gathered together at the dark moon to dream mystical dreams, share wisdom and renew sexual power. Sitting in circle within The Red Tent, they are relieved of their daily responsibilities and cared for by other women. All working and doing aside, together they explore the secrets of the cosmos through the gateway of their wombs. They feed their femininity and emerge refreshed, renewed and empowered by what they have shared and witnessed.

Sisters, it is time to deepen. We will gather together at the dark moon to dream a potent dream of womanhood. We will be fed by the rich stores of nature; nourished by the fullness of our life's journey.

In the warm, cosy space of The Red Tent, you will be nurtured by ancient restorative practices, giving the body, heart, and mind space to rest in stillness, revitalizing your receptivity to life and love. You'll be enchanted by stories, old and new, of Woman and her mysteries. You'll be fed warm soups, vibrant greens, teas: you will be loved from the inside out. You will have the space, the time, the encouragement to simply Be."

Dawn Cartwright, www.chandrabindutantrainstitute.com

OOO

"The dark moon phase, three days a month when we cannot see the moon in our night's sky, was once considered a blessing. In traditional Native American culture, women gathered together in moon lodges … to rest, meditate, heal, let go of the unwanted and celebrate womanhood. They were considered very powerful and they were expected to vision for the whole tribe, helping the Elders with decision making and foresight into the future."

Jane Anderson www.moonandearthconnections.com

Though they are often spoken about interchangeably, it is my understanding that there is a vital difference between a moon lodge and a red tent:

A moon lodge is an introspective experience and one which honours and allows introspective practices: dreaming, trance work, visioning and journaling. It can be undertaken with women together, but is often done alone.

Moon lodges have been in continual use within the Native American tradition for generations, and use distinctive Native American language, myths and austere physical framework. They have been introduced to women in America and beyond in recent years by male chiefs, as well as Susun Weed and her publishing house, Ash Tree.

A red tent is a more communal activity and experience usually in ornate surroundings – one which, whilst allowing for rest and introspection, allows a forum for sharing knowledge, creative activities, ceremony and interaction.

These have been seeded and championed around the US by ALisa Starkweather via the Red Tent Temple movement, as well as independently by a number of other visionary women in the US, Denmark and Australia.

The herstory of the emergence of red tents is being documented in a forthcoming book by ALisa and a film documentary by Isadora Leidenfrost entitled "Things We Don't Talk About: Healing Narratives from the Red Tent".

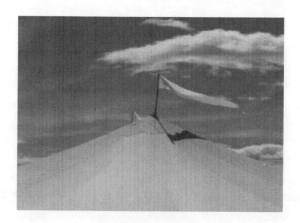

"My heart like yours probably, has been aching when I look into my local area, my world, and see such a great need for the sacred. I see an unmet need in our young to have a place they can count on for mentoring, initiation, and coming into their womanhood with other women. I see an unmet need in our lives to connect deeply, rest and take time to simply be. I see an unmet need for our elders where they can gather to be honoured and share their wisdom.[...] And I wondered what would happen in our societies of local places if women were to have a place we could count on where we are respected, supported and held. I understood from the work that I do that to empower women of any age means to bring health back into a community. And the Red Tent Temple Movement is a means to support us."

> **ALisa Starkweather, at the founding of the Red Tent Temple Movement**

A red tent ...

- *"is part of the spiritual practice of menstruation and the living of the wisdom of the cycles."* **Jane Hardwicke Collings**

- creates a supportive community of women,

- creates a much needed retreat space,

- honours our bodies with time and self-care,

- provides a venue for sharing women's wisdom and celebrating rites of passage,

- creates a woman-centred sacred space within our lives and the world.

The red tent movement seeks to support women around the world in creating sacred places of seclusion where they can take care of themselves during their blood time.

They are springing up around the world in private homes, yurts, festivals and dedicated purpose built rooms. Often draped in red, with beautiful embroidery, fabrics, prayer flags, carpets and paintings, they seek to create a soft, welcoming womb where women can come and speak, cry, sing and laugh, where women share healing, body work, energy work, nourishing meals and herbal tea.

Some temporary red tents have been created for V-day celebrations, art installations and educational projects. Others are more structured women's circles which meet monthly.

They are generally held on the new moon, as this is the traditional time of women's bleeding. But you do not have to be bleeding to go to one, if your own moon time is on a different cycle. The new moon is often a time for sowing the seeds of intentions that we wish to manifest as the moon waxes, so whether or not you are bleeding it is a good time to go.

What happens at a red tent?

"It is very important that we don't shame or hurt one another in the Red Tent Temples by our judgements about what we think "should" happen. With time, with focus, with learning, with dialogue in our circles, with experience, trust that we are going to find our way.

At the same time we help the situation with an orientation sheet about what this is. It helps to invite them into a quiet space. Soft music, a place to close one's eyes and centre, a welcoming that invites each woman to let go of her nervousness, her work, her need to belong and be accepted, and simply come home to herself wherever she is.

It is okay to ask women as they enter to have some quiet time first before getting involved with talking. Talking happens. In the Red Tent in my home, there is quiet talking, nap taking, sometimes tears and often laughter. If you have a crystal bowl or gentle bells that can be struck every once in a while as a way for the room to go within, quiet for a few moments, you can interrupt the pattern in a gentle way of it becoming louder and louder.

Women are not going to be comfortable at first with the idea of doing nothing. I have had very powerful women friends who are very active come into the Red Tent and look like a cat in water. The look says, "what am I doing just sitting here? I should be home DOING something." But that is the point. We are learning the undoing and for that we look like drowned cats momentarily. Soon those same women are stretched out on the pads or receiving energy work or are journaling, sipping tea, and breathing more deeply. It is really a learning experience here."

www.ALisastarkweather.com

Creating a red tent

So you want a red tent for yourself?

Firstly check on-line and in local health food shops or yoga centres to see if there is already one near you. Check the Resources at the end of this book – the groups on Facebook will be able to let you know of any in your area.

If there isn't you will need to brainstorm – perhaps by yourself, or more fun with a few like-minded women.

Grand visioning:
o   Who is it for and why – what is your grandest vision?

o   And what is your simplest first baby step?

o   What do you/ don't you want? What is crucial? What is a deal breaker?

o   What is your one over-riding priority? Community? Retreat? Beauty? This will help to steer you when you feel confused and at sea.

o   What do you like from the pictures and ideas here?

o   What don't you like/want?

Practical visioning:
o   Where to hold it?

o   What date?

o   What time?

o   How long it goes on for.

o   What will you use to decorate it – where will these things come from – use what you have, borrow, get creative refashioning old bits of fabric.

o   Invitation only or posters?

o   Who to invite and do they need to RSVP?

o   What do they bring? Refreshments, cushions…

o   Ensure at least two to set up and two to clear up.

o   Any activities for the tent.

o   Any formal leadership structure.

ALisa Starkweather hosts a monthly teleconference to support women wanting to establish a red tent in their neighbourhood, and is in the process of writing the Red Tent Temple handbook.

Copyright issues and the black and white format of this book prevent me from sharing images of red tents with you. But I urge you to seek them out. There are so many on-line which will, no doubt, inspire you.

Decorating a red tent

Most red tent leaders try to recreate the look and feel of a red tent in an internal room. You can do this with

o   curtains

o   sheets

o   drapes

o   blankets

o   sari fabric

You can get these from:

o   your own cupboards, attics, drawers

o   friends, family and neighbours

o   dye old sheets red

o   buy cheap red sheets from thrift stores, charity shops, retail discounters

o   e-bay has a great choice of very affordable sari fabric - £5 for 5 meters (about $7 for 10 foot)

Or you can have an **actual tent space** – in a **yurt, tepee or a bell tent** (which are much more affordable than yurts, and quicker to put up, but have the same feel) or a cheaper option still, and one which is quick to put up, and can be used inside or out, is a **gazebo** – and you can use it as is or with added drapes.

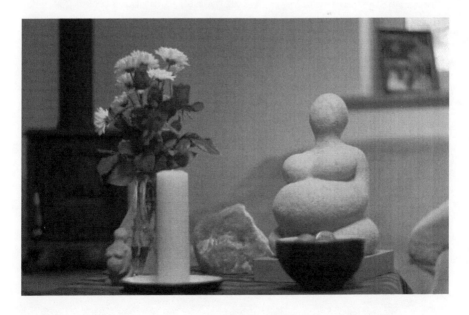

Creating and adorning a space

Equipment you might need includes:

o   Candles, incense, essential oils, smudge stick

o   A portable self-care kit – lavender eye mask, hot water bottle or barley bag, a couple of favourite oils and base oil, a foot-bath

o   A portable shrine or altar – with images of gods/ goddesses/natural items which are meaningful to you and help you to connect with your feeling of sacredness.

o   A creative bag (journal, pens, paints...)

Ensuring your red tent is sustainable

I just want to take a moment, if you are excited about starting a red tent of your own, to caution you to make it sustainable – financially and energetically.

A red tent or any women's group is a labour of love – but should be of many women's love, not just one. Do not work yourself to the bone creating a perfect retreat space for others. After all, you are creating it not just for your community – but for you as well! So ensure that you have support or shared responsibility for:

o   set up

o   clean up

o   finances and administration

o   refreshments

o   hosting

Guidelines for a sustainable red tent

o Do not do it all yourself and wear yourself out. Allow others to help in serving your community, and in serving **you**!

o Don't worry about making it perfect. Just make it with love, and aim for beauty and it will be wonderful. Consider it a work in progress which will grow with you all, using the skills and energy of all its members – as it sustains you, so you sustain it.

o Get support and advice from other women who have gone before you – join an online group or take part in the Red Tent Temple teleconferences.

o Ensure your decorations are quick, or at least pleasurable, to set up!

o Make sure not to try to cram in too many activities or ideas – remember first and foremost a red tent is a place to **be**.

o Be gentle with yourself in its creation. There are many who may sneer or denigrate your sacred project. I have many of these people around me. They do not need to know, whilst you still feel tender and vulnerable. If you feel concerned, keep it private and discrete.

o It is a sacred space, share it with only those who will honour it as such. Request at the beginning of each session that women let what emerges in the tent, to stay in the tent – ensuring the emotional safety of all who enter it.

o Be clear on how new women are invited. Will you put up posters, or simply have it amongst a closed group of friends? If it is in a person's home then the size of room, and people's privacy might demand that it is invitation only and that people RSVP.

The more sustainable your red tent is, the longer it will be there to support you and your community.

Creating your own moon lodge

The original moon lodge consisted of a woven hazel branch frame with a cover made of hides, blankets or cloth – a similar type of construction to a sweat lodge. They tend to be much simpler and less ornate than red tent spaces.

I have visions of creating a moon lodge in the tea house where this book was written, and where I was married. It is a beautiful hand-constructed space nestled in the woods with thick plastered walls, a thatched roof, round fire place and panoramic views over the marsh and sea. Being just one room it feels like a safe womb. It smells of sweet cedar and incense. There are lots of big cushions, comfy chairs and warm woollen blankets. In short it spells comfort and retreat for me. But when I can't get there in person, I recreate this feeling in my bedroom at home.

A dear friend is creating a moon lodge in an abandoned woodland hut. She will let other trusted women know of this space, so that they too can retreat to it when they need.

Lodges which are used by many women often keep a lodge book where any woman can share her insights, visions or dreams – these may support another woman in her own process, as well as give material for contemplation.

OOO

Most of us do not (yet!) have a moon lodge or red tent space in our neighbourhoods. And for many of us our moon time is private – we have no desire to step outside our front doors or be sociable.

Perhaps setting up a red tent is not for you, or not feasible right now. Perhaps you do not yet have a circle of likeminded women to share in creating one. Perhaps you feel like you do not have the resources. Or perhaps you just need the courage to act on your dreams.

We are the ones we've be waiting for!

AFTERWORD

Dearest moon sisters – have fun creating your own special spaces and ceremonies – be they public or private, intricate or simple. I would love to know how you get on – do send me your stories and pictures! It is my wish that a future edition of this book will share all of your beautiful examples from around the world, to inspire another generation of women to create spaces to honour their female selves and retreat. I would love to hear your insights and responses to this book and to see your creations. You can email me at **lucy@thehappywomb.com**

What a journey this has been for me, and for you too I hope! What learning, what courage and insight we have unearthed on our travels together. What wisdom we have in our bodies and in ancient women's cultures that we can bring into our lives today.

Thank you for your companionship on the journey. I wish you well as you travel onwards.

If you have enjoyed this book do consider buying one for friends, daughters or sisters. And please join me at **www.thehappywomb.com** for a whole host of Woman-craft resources.

Blessings to you.

Lucy Pearce,

Cork, Ireland, January 2012.

RESOURCES

This list is by no means exhaustive, but I have found them to be of use both in my personal life and in researching this book.

On-line resources
Charting

www.menstruation.com.au/fertility/example.html - *Example of fertility chart*

www.menstruation.com.au/fertility/mychart.html - *Blank fertility chart*

www.menstruation.com.au/menstrualproducts/hormonalforecaster.html - *Free fertility predictor software*

www.thebillingsovulationmethod.org *Fertility awareness from the original discoverers of The Ovulation Method – free e-books and charts (go to their resources section)*

Sources of moon diaries and charts

www.wemoon.ws

www.earthpathwaysdiary.co.uk

www.earthlightcollective.com *for beautiful annotated and illustrated moon dial mandalas* www.moontimes.co.uk *for moon bracelets, dials, diaries and calendars:*

www.herbalmedicinehealing.com

www.moonandearthconnections.com

Leading women in the field of menstrual education

www.womensquest.org – Alexandra Pope

www.mirandagray.co.uk – Miranda Gray

www.alisastarkweather.com -ALisa Starkweather

www.deannalam.com – DeAnna L'am

www.moonsong.com.au – Jane Hardwicke Collings

Personal blogs which celebrate moon time

dreamingaloudnet.blogspot.com

meztlicihuatl-english.blogspot.com

aiyanawoman.blogspot.com/2010/09/red-tents-and-bleeding-cycles.html

lorithemidwife.wordpress.com

redtenttempleatmotherroots.blogspot.com

spiraltraditions.blogspot.com

www.ShawnDellJoyce.com

janehardwickecollings-moonsong.blogspot.com

Woman Honouring websites

www.thehappywomb.com

www.dreamingaloud.net

www.optimizedwoman.com

www.wombyoga.org

www.chandrabindutantrainstitute.com

www.crimsonwisdom.com

www.redwebfoundation.org

www.yoni.com

www.onewoman.com

www.menstruation.com

www.goddessguidebook.com

www.crimsoncampaign.org

Mothers and daughters

www.moonandearthconnections.com/menstruationbooklets.htm - *for the text of a whole menarche book on-line*

www.moontimes.co.uk *– stocks a good number of independently published guides on menarche*

www.joyw.org/redthreadcircles.htm *place for mother and daughters to connect through community and creativity*

www.theredboxcompany.com *for gifts and free menarche resources*

Red tents and moon lodges

www.alisastarkweather.com - *for detailed insight in to the "what" and "how" of red tents this is the best resource I have found. ALisa founded the grassroots Red Tent Temple Movement in 2007 that is spreading round the world.*

www.redtenttemplemovement.com - *a grassroots movement aiming to bring a red tent to every neighborhood. They hold a monthly teleconference to support women in getting started.*

www.redtentmovie.com - *This visually stunning film is directed and produced by women features red tents all over the US. It will be released later in 2012. Trailers can now be seen on the website. 10% of the income from the e-version of this book and my Red Tent guide will be donated to the project.*

www.sacredmoon.com.au

www.theredtent.net

Facebook community pages

Red Tent Movement

Red tents Moon lodges Red tent temples

Women's Red Tents and Temples Worldwide

Red Tent Film

Red Tents in Every Neighbourhood

The Moon Woman

The Happy Womb

Dreaming Aloud

<u>Red Tent Videos on-line</u>

Introduction to red tents and celebrating menarche

http://youtube/1enWN7n8l3E

A Red Tent being set up in a living room

http://youtube/nnFjMlxui7o

DeAnna L'am's Red Tent in California

http://www.youtube.com/watch?v=CQ39pZC6DRs
http://wn.com/The_Red_Tent

Books

Moon Time

Red Moon: Understanding and using the creative sexual and spiritual gifts of the menstrual cycle – Miranda Gray

The Red Tent – Anita Diamant

Thirteen Moons – Rachael Hertogs *(available from www.moontimes.co.uk) full of goddess wisdom, astrology, Native American wisdom, reusable sanitary protection and articles from most of the major authors noted here. A compendium of women's wisdom.*

The Wise Wound – Penelope Shuttle & Peter Redgrave

Your Body Speaks Your Mind – D. Shapiro

Grandmother Moon: Lunar Magic In Our Lives-Spells, Rituals, Goddesses, Legends and Emotions – Z. Budapest.

Women Circling the Earth - Beverley Engle

Sister Moon Lodge: The Power and the Mystery of Menstruation - Stepanich Kisma

The Optimized Woman - Miranda Gray

Her Blood is Gold: Celebrating the Power of Menstruation – Lara Owen

Honoring Menstruation: A Time of Self-Renewal – Lara Owen

Songs of Bleeding – Spider

Menarche

Menarche: A Journey into Womanhood – Rachael Hertogs *(available from www.moontimes.co.uk)*

Celebrating Girls – Virginia Beane-Rutter

A Blessing not a Curse: A mother daughter guide to the transition from child to woman – Jane Bennett

A Diva's Guide to Getting Your First Period – DeAnna L'am with gloriously creative and bright illustrations by Jessica Jarman-Hayes

Moon Mother, Moon Daughter – Janet Lucy & Terri Allison

Puberty Girl – Shushann Movsessian

The Thundering Years: Rituals and Sacred Wisdom for Teens – Julie Tallard Johnson

The Seven Sacred Rites of Menarche – Kristi Meisenbach Boylan

First Moon – Maureen Theresa Smith

Becoming Peers – DeAnna L'am

Becoming a Woman: A Guide for Girls Approaching Menstruation – Jane Hardwicke Collings

A Time To Celebrate: A Celebration of a Girl's First Menstrual Period –
Joan Morais

Reviving Ophelia – Mary Pipher

Mother-Daughter Wisdom: Understanding the Crucial Links Between Mothers, Daughters and Health – Dr Christiane Northrup

Women's herbals

Herbal Healing for Women – Rosemary Gladstar

Neal's Yard Natural Remedies – Susan Curtis

Holistic Women's Herbal – K Campion

Wise Womans' Herbal for the Childbearing Year – Susun Weed

Women's health

Women's Bodies, Women's Wisdom – Dr Christiane Northrup

Woman's Health in Woman's Hands – D. Cooper

New Menopausal Years: The Wise Woman W – Alternative Approaches for Women 30–90 – Susun Weed.

The Pill: Are you sure it's for you? – Jane Bennett and Alexandra Pope

Taking charge of your fertility – Toni Weschler

Read my Lips: A Complete Guide to the Vagina and Vulva – Debbie Herbenick & Vanessa Schick

Yoni Shakti Tantra: the thinking woman's guide to freedom – Uma Dinsmore Tuli

Self-care

Succulent Wild Woman: Dancing with your wonder-full self – SARK

You Can Heal Your Life – Louise. L. Hay

The Woman's Comfort Book – Jennifer Louden

The Woman's Retreat Book – Jennifer Louden

Women's Wisdom

Maps to Ecstasy: The Healing Power of Movement – Gabrielle Roth

Circle of Stones – Judith Duerk

73 Lessons Every Goddess Must Know – Goddess Leonie Dawson

Succulent Wild Woman: Dancing with Your Wonder Full Self – SARK

Women Who Run with the Wolves – Clarissa Pinkola Estes

Ix Chel Wisdom – Shonagh Home (from www.shonaghhome.com)

Keys to the Open Gate: A Woman's Spirituality Sourcebook – Kimberley Snow

The Woman's Quest – Unfolding Women's Path of Power and Wisdom – Alexandra Pope (from www.wildgenie.com)

The Vagina Monologues – Eve Ensler

Bodies – Susie Orbach

She Walks in Beauty – A Woman's Journey Through Poems – selected by Caroline Kennedy

Herstory – free e-book of women's history available from www.moonsong.com.au

ABOUT THE AUTHOR

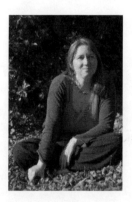

Lucy Pearce is a teacher of Woman-craft and creativity and a women's group founder. She is mama to three young children and lives on the East Cork coast in Ireland.

She works as a free-spirited freelance writer and is a regular contributor to *Modern Mum* magazine, *The Irish Examiner* and JUNO magazine, where her column, Dreaming Aloud, has run since 2009. On-line she contributes to *Rhythm of the Home*, *The Anti-Room* and *Wild Sister* magazine. She is contributing editor at JUNO.

This is her first book. She is currently working on her second about Creative Rainbow Mothers.

She blogs at **www.dreamingaloud.net** on living philosophy, moon time, everyday zen and gentle parenting. Her website **www.thehappywomb.com** features Woman-craft: honouring moon time, women's circles, creativity, rites of passage, natural pregnancy, holistic birth preparation and so much more. Lucy is available to facilitate workshops and for speaking engagements. Contact her at **lucy@thehappywomb.com**

This book can be purchased as an e-book from The HappyWomb.com. The e-book has a printable moon dial and is more comprehensively illustrated, including images of red tents.

Shorter e-booklets containing excerpted material from the original *Moon Time* e-book are also available:

- **Menarche: Celebrating a girl's first period**
  (25 A4 pages)
- **Positively Menstrual: Natural healing for PMT**
  (32 A4 pages)
- **Red Tents and Moon Lodges: Creating sacred female space for moon time retreat**
  (23 A4 pages)

✓ Highly practical guides, full of ideas and approaches from a veteran woman's group facilitator.
✓ Tailored specifically to your needs – just get the information you need!
✓ Ready to print PDF format.
✓ Illustrated with inspiringly beautiful colour photography.
✓ With a comprehensive resource section at the back for web and book resources.

Coming soon, from the same author –
The Moods of Motherhood
and
How to Be a Creative Rainbow Mama!